D0754028

Essential Oils *of the* Bible

RANDI MINETOR

Essential Oils *of the* Bible

Connecting God's Word to Natural Healing

ALTHEA
PRESS

For general information on our other products and services or to obtain technical support, please contact our Customer Care Department within the United States at (866) 744-2665, or outside the United States at (510) 253-0500.

Althea Press publishes its books in a variety of electronic and print formats. Some content that appears in print may not be available in electronic books, and vice versa.

TRADEMARKS: Althea Press and the Althea Press logo are trademarks or registered trademarks of Callisto Media Inc. and/or its affiliates, in the United States and other countries, and may not be used without written permission. All other trademarks are the property of their respective owners. Althea Press is not associated with any product or vendor mentioned in this book.

Illustrations by Tom Bingham © 2016; stained glass © Vertyr/Shutterstock; p. 16, 21, 29 courtesy of archive.org (archive.org/details/lifeofourlordsav00flee; archive.org/details/pictorialbibleco00cobb); back cover photograph © Kristin Rogers Photography/Stocksy, front cover photographs © Shutterstock

ISBN: Print 978-1-62315-738-8 | eBook 978-1-62315-739-5

To Gabrielle, Carlo, Dustin, and Christina

Contents

Introduction

IN GENESIS 28, Jacob made camp on his way to a new home in Padanaram. He laid his head on a stone to sleep, and he had a dream.

" . . . and behold a ladder set up on the earth, and the top of it reached to heaven: and behold the angels of God ascending and descending on it," the record tells us. "And behold the Lord stood above it, and said, 'I am the Lord God of Abraham thy father, and the God of Isaac.'"

Jacob awoke and said, "Surely the Lord is in this place; and I knew it not." He got to work piling up the stones on which he had slept, forming them into a pillar—"and poured oil upon the top of it." Jacob then swore an oath: " . . . this stone, which I have set for a pillar, shall be God's house."

This is the first Biblical record of the practice of anointment, the pouring of oil over an object or a person to consecrate it in the eyes of God. Anointment is mentioned repeatedly in the Bible, and, today, priests and ministers still anoint people at moments in their lives that involve their commitment to God. While the old method involved pouring a vessel of oil over a person's head, priests today usually use a drop of oil on a thumb to form the sign of the cross on a person's forehead.

Today's anointing oil often contains the scents used in preparations for the first holy temple—the ones specified by God to Moses for the holy anointing oil and the holy incense. Myrrh, galbanum, onycha, frankincense, cinnamon, calamus, and cassia all find their way into religious use.

We can use these scents—as well as many others noted in the Bible—in our own homes and enjoy the same healing properties that people of ancient times discovered and passed down through generations. Essential oils are widely available to anyone who would like to make a deeper connection with the stories of the Bible.

Let me say that I am a person of both faith and science; I see the parallels between God's work and man's discovery, and I believe these work in tandem to create the wonders that are the Earth and the universe. This is the appeal of essential oils for me—they, too, are grounded in both science and faith. Scientific evidence tells us that many of these oils are as effective as pharmaceuticals in easing pain and suffering, while faith tells us these connections to the natural world go back thousands of years, and that God intended them to be so.

We can use these scents and enjoy the same healing properties that people of ancient times discovered and passed down through generations.

I have used lavender and tea tree essential oils to calm anxiety, take the sting out of sunburn, and remove the "little things" that appear on skin as we pass middle age. When colds and flu strike, I turn to eucalyptus and spearmint essential oils.

I hope you find this book useful in creating a lasting connection between your own home and family and the words of God. Be inspired, and be healed.

CHAPTER ONE

The Sacred Link of Essential Oils

With my holy oil have
I anointed him.

—PSALM 89:20

God spoke these words as He declared His protection of David, naming him a prophet and king of the people of Israel. Once anointed, David encountered many difficulties and challenges to his authority, but no one could depose him or harm him in any lasting way. The simple act of anointment—in this case, directly from God—shielded him from every adversary for the rest of his days.

What was this gift of oil that God bestowed on David, and was it reserved for a chosen few? By the time David became king, oils had been a mainstay of spirituality and healing for thousands of years. As each successive generation understood the value of oils to their health and well-being, plants that produced oil became so valuable that Pharisees in Jesus Christ's day required people to turn over 10 percent—a tax system known as tithing—of the oil-producing herbs and spices they cultivated.

Today, the oils from these plants are bottled as essential oils, and you can build a personal apothecary to treat everything from a scraped knee to the pain of arthritis. Just as the Bible tells us, we can use essential oils to become closer to God, and to return to natural methods of healing in our everyday lives.

The Bible, Personal and Present

You may be reading this book because you would like to take advantage of all the natural power of essential oils, and because you want to form a stronger bond between your family and your faith. Or perhaps you feel comfortable with your personal relationship with God, but seek additional ways to express it—not just for yourself, but for your spouse and children, as well.

Many people feel this powerful link with their faith and with God, but they feel less connected to the Bible and its many teachings. We reference the familiar stories instantly: Joseph's rise to power in Canaan even as his brothers betrayed him; Moses leading his people out of Egypt; King Solomon's courting of and marriage to the daughter of Pharaoh and the trouble that followed their nuptials; Job's devastating losses at the whims of God and Satan; and, of course, the stories of Jesus and his disciples as they made their way to Gethsemane and Christ's eventual fate. We've heard the stories since childhood, but it may be rare that we actually pick up the Bible and explore them again.

In the bustle of twenty-first-century life, sitting with the Bible on a daily basis can be a luxury of time most people cannot afford. Tasks at work and at home crowd our schedules, making even a few minutes of Bible study impractical at best. The digital world has changed our relationship with the Bible, as well; today we can search any translation of the Bible, using keywords to find exactly the story or message we need, and thereby limiting the possibilities of discovering a related passage that may bring a helpful or enlightening verse we actually need even more.

So what do we do? How can we reinforce our values and emulate the behavior God endorses in the Bible, even if we have little time to set aside for studying Scripture?

Many people find a strengthened connection to the Bible and to God through essential oils, by making the scents and therapeutic properties of these oils a part of daily life.

The benefits of these oils go well beyond their pleasant scents. They provided people of ancient times with the tools they needed to tend to the sick, purify their homes, and keep themselves free of pain and disease. As you develop your own uses for essential oils, you will forge a deeper connection with the Bible, one founded by putting God's word into practice and using the tools He provides in medicinal plants from around the world.

Please note: In this book, I have quoted chapters and verses from the King James Version of the Bible, still the most popular Bible in print. When later translations changed the names of some of the plants (for example, as the reference in Isaiah 41:19 to the shittah tree in King James became "acacia" in the New International Version and subsequent translations), I have noted this in the description of the essential oil in chapter 3. Most of these changes do not change the meaning, and simply put a modern name on a plant of ancient times.

The Power of Anointment

The most familiar use of oils in the Bible is in ceremonies of anointment, whether it be an altar or tabernacle, a dishful of wafers, or the head and feet of Christ. In the Old Testament, to be anointed—especially in carrying out God's instruction to do so—gave a person, a building, or an object the divine protection of the Lord.

In the Bible, God directs His people to combine specific oils, spices, and herbs and use them to consecrate the first holy sanctuary, making the scent of this sacred blend part of the experience upon entering the temple. So it was that essential oils became part of religious life from the very beginning of the Judeo-Christian tradition. Anointment with such oils, however, was reserved for very special ceremonies, including the consecration of high priests and kings. We find evidence of more everyday uses in Christ's time, all of which we'll explore in the pages that follow.

Biblical Anointment

Many of these stories may be familiar to you, but how much do you know about the practice of anointing, and the oils used for the ceremonies? By looking at a few episodes of anointment discussed in the Bible, we can learn about the importance of this ritual to the earliest Jews and Christians.

THE OLD TESTAMENT

The Old Testament contains seven episodes of one person anointing another, each of which gave the anointed one stature and authority.

In Exodus 29:7–21, God directed Moses to bring his older brother, Aaron, to the tabernacle they had built—also according to God's specific instructions—and to anoint Aaron, making him the first high priest of the Jewish people. "Then shalt thou take the anointing oil, and pour it upon his head, and anoint him," God said, and then told them to kill a ram and spill its blood on the altar. "And thou shalt take of the blood that is upon the altar, and of the anointing oil, and sprinkle it upon Aaron, and upon his garments, and upon his sons, and upon the garments of his sons with him; and he shall be hallowed, and his garments, and his sons, and his sons' garments with him."

In 1 Samuel 10:1, Samuel anointed Saul—a young man from Gibeah who happened on Samuel while looking for his family's donkeys—as the reluctant leader of the Israelites. Saul's reign did not go smoothly, however, and in 1 Samuel 16:12–13, Samuel anointed David of Jesse as the next leader in Israel. In 2 Samuel 2:4, he anointed David once again, this time placing him over the house of Judah; in 2 Samuel 5:3, David was anointed by Samuel a third time, making him king of Israel.

When next we hear of anointing, however, it took place during a personal trial: King David, as told in 2 Samuel 12, fasted and prayed for seven days while his infant child lay on the verge of death. When servants finally informed him that the child had died, David "arose from the earth, and washed, and anointed himself, and changed his apparel, and came into the house of the Lord, and worshipped. . . ."

Here, 2 Samuel gives us a glimpse of anointing as part of everyday life in Biblical times, a way of using oil to cleanse oneself after the death of a loved one.

We do not hear of other anointments in the Bible until Ezekiel 16:9: "Then washed I thee with water; yea, I thoroughly washed away thy blood from thee, and I anointed thee with oil." Here, anointment becomes a metaphor for God's care of Israel in the wilderness during the time of Moses. In this and all other references to anointment in the Bible, we find that the practice had become part of any number of cleansing rituals, whether they were performed by kings, the working class, or the poor in the streets of ancient cities.

THE NEW TESTAMENT

By the time we begin the New Testament, we find that anointing had become commonplace, an act that any person could perform—but doing so still carried with it a measure of holiness and honor. In Mark 6:13, Jesus and his apostles went to the poor and sick and anointed them, using this practice as a method of healing. In Mark 14:3–8, a woman "having an alabaster box of ointment of spikenard very precious" anointed Jesus by pouring the expensive oil over his head. When people around him objected that the oil could have been sold to benefit the poor, Jesus told them, "Ye have the poor with you always, and whensoever ye will ye may do them good: but me ye have not always. She hath done what she could: she is come aforehand to anoint my body to the burying."

In Luke 7:36–47, a woman who was a known sinner came to the home of a Pharisee where Jesus had been invited to take a meal. As he ate, she washed his feet with her own tears, wiped them dry with her hair, and anointed his feet with the ointment she had brought in an alabaster box. The Pharisee objected that Jesus should not allow such a sinner to touch him, but Jesus told him, "I entered into thine house, thou gavest me no water for my feet; but she hath washed my feet with tears, and wiped them with the hairs of her head. . . . Her sins, which are many, are forgiven; for she loved much: but he who is forgiven little, loves little."

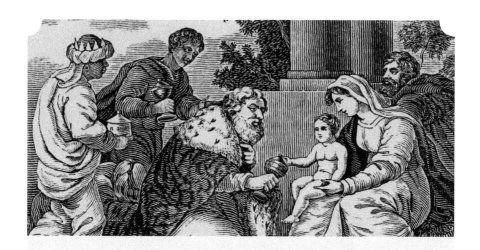

THE GIFTS OF THE MAGI

In Matthew 2:11, we learn of the wise men who came to Bethlehem to see the young child Jesus at home with Mary and Joseph, and to worship him, bringing him three gifts: gold, frankincense, and myrrh. In the eyes of modern readers, the spices seem like odd gifts to bring any child—but Biblical history tells us otherwise.

Myrrh was one of the chief ingredients in the holy anointing oil that God commanded Moses to make in Exodus 30:23; a few verses later, when God gave Moses the recipe for the holy incense that would scent the first great temple, He told Moses to combine "these sweet spices with pure frankincense." Both spices have value in healing, as well: relieving pain, reducing swelling, killing viruses and fungal infections, and keeping wounds from becoming septic or infected. Myrrh even has the added benefit of aiding in sleep, while frankincense helps open breathing passages and clear phlegm from the chest and lungs. Mary and Joseph would have appreciated the wise men's thoughtfulness and generosity in bringing gifts of such practical value to the newborn Jesus and his family.

Anointment Today

What do all these stories tell us about the way we should practice everyday anointment today? Anointing in the early days of the Bible set these people apart in their service to God and to their fellow human beings, a special honor using oils and spices very dear to the people of the time. In the New Testament, however, Jesus and his apostles used oils to protect and heal the sick, and for cleansing, while others brought oils to Jesus as a demonstration of their love for him.

It's not likely that most people today have the opportunity to anoint a king or a priest, but we certainly can consider our use of essential oils as a practice to protect and hallow someone in the eyes of God—essentially, to bring them to God's notice for special consideration. A loved one who is ill, for example, may be a focus of your prayers, making him an appropriate candidate for anointment with fragrant oils. A new beginning such as a first communion, the first night in a new home, or the start of a long journey may be the impetus to anoint a dear friend, a family member, or a neighbor, and to mark the event with a prayer as well. Priests and ministers of many churches use bedside anointment as part of the last rites.

Many churches believe that the anointing oil symbolizes the Holy Spirit, and that the brief ceremony of anointment, coupled with prayer, releases the Holy Spirit so it may do its work. That said, anointment should never be a complete substitute for medical intervention—the work of modern medicine is part of God's creation, and should be accepted as one of the gifts he gives us to cure sickness and heal injury.

How to anoint? In the Bible, oil runs down Aaron's robes as Moses pours it over his head, but this is not practical in most modern settings. Here are some basic guidelines:

1. Use olive oil. Olive oil has the greatest connection to Biblical oil, as it was the most-available oil in the days of the Old and New Testaments.
2. Choose the essential oils that you prefer. Select any scented oils you wish to include, based on the information you will find in chapter 3.

3. Pour 2 tablespoons of olive oil into a small, dark amber or cobalt glass bottle, and then add 1 to 2 drops of each of the essential oils you have chosen.
4. Say a prayer over the oil. The prayer is of your own choosing—there is no set text for this—but it should ask for God's blessing of purity for the oil.
5. To anoint yourself or a loved one, place a drop of the oil on your thumb. Make the sign of the cross on the forehead of the person you are anointing. As you do this, say, "I anoint you in the name of the Father, and the Son, and the Holy Spirit, amen."
6. Continue with a prayer that is appropriate to the specific circumstance. For example, you may pray for the health of a sick person, or for God's blessing for a child starting her first day of school, or for blessings and a good life for a couple in their first home.
7. Store any unused oil in a cool, dark place out of the sun, for example, in a closet or in a box with other essential oils.

Oils in the Bible

Regardless of your denomination, you know that frankincense and myrrh figure prominently at the outset of Jesus's life—but you may not be aware of the many other spices, herbs, and plants that produced essential oils in Biblical times. In fact, at least 30 plants produced oil, resin, or sap that was used in homes and houses of worship. We know this because they are named throughout the Bible, in both the Old and New Testaments.

The balm of Gilead, for example, was distilled from the balsam fir, a tree that grows abundantly in the Middle East, as well as in Europe and North America. Calamus, also known as sweet flag, was one of the plant substances God told Moses to include in the holy anointing oil. Mint, anise, and rue are all mentioned in the Gospels as plants so valuable that the Pharisees determined they must be tithed. And myrtle, valued for its tensile strength as well as for its astringent properties, was one of the materials God specified for the building of huts during the annual Feast of Tabernacles.

Today we can take the essences of these plants and use them in their most concentrated form, making the most of their powers in aromatherapy, cleansing, and natural healing.

Essential Oils

Essential oils are the true essence of a plant. They come from a group of molecules in plants called terpenes (or hydrocarbons), the substances that create the plant's scent. Each plant has a unique combination of terpenes, so the scent of that plant is unique—and each plant has its own set of benefits that differs from any other plant.

*And he made the holy anointing oil,
and the pure incense of sweet spices,
according to the work of the apothecary.*

—EXODUS 37:29

The use of these plants for healing likely began even before the Bible brings them into its narrative. The results of trial and error were passed down verbally from generation to generation until they could be recorded in writing, and as techniques for extracting the essences of the plants became more available, the uses for each plant increased.

Essential oils are mentioned nearly 200 times in the Bible, many of them in relation to specific uses already in common practice. (You'll find a list of citations in Scripture toward the end of the book, on page 203.) People used these oils as medicine to ward off infection and treat illnesses and wounds, as well as to induce sleep, cleanse their homes and bodies, honor a visitor, and show devotion to another person.

Today we use many of these essential oils in the same ways they were used in the Bible. Further exploration, including a wealth of contributions by science, has shown us a wider variety of ways we can put these oils to use, and the safest and most effective ways to use them.

The following is a list of the 30 essential oils mentioned in the Bible and examined in detail in chapter 3. In some cases, you will see the modern name for this oil in parentheses after the Biblical name.

- Aloes (Sandalwood)
- Anise
- Balm (Balsam)
- Bay (Bay laurel)
- Bdellium
- Calamus
- Camphire (Henna)
- Cassia
- Cedar (Cedarwood)
- Cinnamon
- Coriander
- Cumin
- Cypress
- Fir
- Frankincense
- Galbanum
- Hyssop
- Juniper
- Mint (Spearmint)
- Mustard seed
- Myrrh
- Myrtle
- Onycha (Benzoin)
- Pine
- Rose of Sharon (Cistus/Rock rose)
- Rue
- Saffron
- Shittah (Acacia, Gum arabic)
- Spikenard
- Wormwood

Olive Oil

Essential oils and the plants from which they originate are not the only oils mentioned in the Bible. Other plants provided oils that served a wide range of purposes, from lamp fuel to lubricants for hair and skin.

In Exodus 27:20, as part of His detailed instructions for the building of the first great temple, God tells Moses to "command the children of Israel, that they bring thee pure oil olive beaten for the light, to cause the lamp to burn always." In this way God told the Jewish people to keep an eternal flame burning in houses of worship, an instruction that rabbis follow to this day.

Olive oil is not an essential oil but it became a staple in Biblical times as a much-prized commodity that landowners grew and produced in abundance. Kings kept storehouses filled with vessels of olive oil, and communities stored the valuable oil against the possibility of years of famine, when the trees might not bear fruit. So ubiquitous was this oil to the people of the Bible that they named

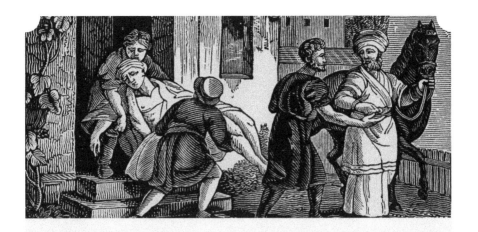

THE HEALING HAND OF GOD

A certain man went down from Jerusalem to Jericho, and
fell among thieves, which stripped him of his raiment, and
wounded him, and departed, leaving him half dead. . . . But
a certain Samaritan, as he journeyed, came where he was:
and when he saw him, he had compassion on him, and went
to him, and bound up his wounds, pouring in oil and wine,
and set him on his own beast, and brought him to an inn, and
took care of him.—Luke 10:30–34

Jesus tells the story of the Good Samaritan to illustrate the concept
of looking out for our neighbors as well as ourselves, but, as in all of
his parables, he chose his words carefully. Pouring oil on the beaten
man's wounds was instrumental in his survival, and Jesus noted its
use as an illustration of the good we can do when we show kindness
and mercy to others. Oil, in this case, begins the healing process
that continues as the Samaritan takes care of the man he saved.

When essential oils are combined with loving care, they can be part
of the greater good we bring to others.

a mountain the Mount of Olives, locating their olive presses at the foot of the incline to take best advantage of the many groves of olive trees there. There, Jesus spent his last evening as a free man, in the garden of Gethsemane—a Hebrew name that means "press of oil."

Today, medical science tells us that olive oil is one of the healthiest oils to use in our diet because it is loaded with monounsaturated fat, which promotes the good HDL cholesterol for cardiovascular health. We also use it as a carrier oil, an oil that retains its liquid form when heated, making it a stable carrier for essential oils. In chapter 2, you will learn about combining essential oils with a carrier oil of your choice to make these oils safe to apply topically to the body.

Faith and Faithful Practice

By learning how essential oils were used in the Bible, we can become more in touch with our faith, and feel closer to God and Christ as we use the essential oils in our everyday lives. We can be guided by the sense of doing what Jesus and the apostles did to heal the sick and wounded, and by what God commanded when He gave instructions for building the first house of worship.

That said, we must be mindful that God does not simply grant wishes. Faith alone cannot guarantee healing, and the use of essential oils may not always be enough to ward off anxiety, cure illness, or protect against disease. God sees a much larger and more intricate picture than we can possibly imagine, and our role in that picture may not be exactly what we hope it will be.

While we can't know what God has in store for us, we do know this: Faith makes us stronger. When you use your essential oils, bring your faith into the process of mixing and administering them. Just as you might reach out to God before going into an important meeting or as your child begins a championship soccer game, make this same connection as you use your essential oils. Whatever the outcome, you will know that God is with you, and that He heard your prayer and guided your hand.

Thou preparest a table before me in the presence of mine enemies: thou anointest my head with oil; my cup runneth over.

—PSALMS 23:5

How to Use This Book

Why a book about essential oils in the Bible? This book brings to light an aspect of Scripture you may never have considered before— one that can have a practical application in your daily life. In all the ways we hope to achieve a deeper connection to God and Christ, this book provides a practical way to do so today, while adding the natural healing properties and pleasing scents of essential oils to your family's life.

In the chapters that follow, you'll find an introduction to essential oils and how they work. Profiles of the essential oils used in Biblical times will help you understand their significance; the recipes in chapter 4 provide remedies for everyday ailments that make the most of the versatility of essential oils, both those specified in the Bible and other essential oils now in common use. Today we have many more oils available to us than the people of Biblical times did, so we can draw on the world's variety for healing, cleansing, scenting, and many other applications, in every aspect of our lives.

CHAPTER TWO

How Essential Oils Heal

*Is any sick among
you? Let him call for the
elders of the church,
and let them pray over
him, anointing him with oil
in the name of the Lord.*

—JAMES 5:14

God has provided the natural power of essential oils for our use in a wide range of applications, and He made it possible for our distant ancestors to discover these natural resources in their own environments. Essential oils not only have healing power, but they also have staying power; many of the oils cited in the Bible are still in common use today.

Why is this? Scientific research has shown us that these oils contain hydrocarbons—the same compounds that produce their unique scents—that promote healing and wellness. In fact, some of these oils are as effective as their pharmaceutical counterparts in treating non-life-threatening conditions and illnesses.

In this chapter, we'll talk about the safe use of essential oils, the tools you need to use your oils effectively, and the ingenuity built into God's creations.

The Healing Power of Essential Oils

Some essential oils are *adaptogens*—substances that help us adapt to environmental factors that cause stress, and reduce the potential for damage caused by these stressors. Most adaptogens are naturally occurring, and a number of them—especially herbs grown in India—have been in use by medical practitioners for thousands of years.

Many essential oils can be either calming or stimulating, depending on the body's need to deal with stress. For example, one person may find the scent of lavender essential oil to be calming and uplifting on a day filled with petty annoyances. Another person may use the same lavender scent to re-energize after a virtually sleepless night at home with a new baby. The essential oil literally adapts to the situation, giving the body what it needs to face the challenge.

The following list of essential oils with adaptogenic properties will help you choose the right one for your home or workplace.

- **Bergamot:** This essential oil mellows and uplifts, making it useful for anxiety, depression, stress, and even anorexia.

- **Cedarwood:** The fresh, clean scent acts to calm anxiety and relieve tension.

- **German Chamomile:** This oil relieves the pain and tension of menstrual and menopausal symptoms, making it a woman's lifelong remedy.

- **Roman Chamomile:** Agitation and PMS are two of this oil's targets.

- **Frankincense:** For agitation, anxiety, skin inflammation, and stress, there's no essential oil that's more versatile.

- **Geranium:** In addition to its medicinal powers, geranium relieves stress and PMS.

- **Jasmine:** Depression and anxiety ease with the use of this oil.

- **Lavender:** The single most versatile essential oil, lavender fights anxiety, tension, stress, insomnia, and just about every other tension-related ailment.

- **Peppermint:** This essential oil relieves depression and mental fatigue, fights stress, and eases away migraines and other headaches.

- **Sandalwood:** Relief from depression, stress, and tension are just a few of this oil's many attributes.

. . . for so were the days of their purifications accomplished, to wit, six months with oil of myrrh, and six months with sweet odours, and with other things for the purifying of the women.

—ESTHER 2:12

The Benefits of Using Essential Oils

We so often feel helpless when we or our loved ones are ill or in pain, and the means that most of us have available to combat common ailments can be limited. With our personal apothecary of essential oils, however, we have the tools to make a difference—both in treating the symptoms and in creating a calming, pain-reducing atmosphere.

- **Essential oils are completely natural.** Most are steam distilled or cold pressed from the plants, so the oils contain nothing but the plant's essence. No chemicals are involved; each bottle provides only the purest ingredients found in nature.

- **Essential oils can bring peace, calm, and focus in a hectic world.** The naturally occurring volatile organic compounds (VOCs) in essential oils have beneficial effects on the mind as well as the body, gently clearing your head and calming your nerves.

- **Essential oils have a long shelf life.** When properly stored (see page 32, "Getting Started with Essential Oils"), essential oils can provide months or years of use at their full strength. Compare this with similarly priced OTC analgesics and other remedies, many of which expire in a year or less.

- **Essential oils are affordable.** The ones you will use most often tend to be the most reasonably priced—and while a few oils require a significant investment, you can substitute less expensive choices for the most costly oils.

- **Essential oils are versatile.** Each has a wide variety of uses, and you can mix several together to multiply the benefits. Chapter 4 provides many recipes that address all kinds of ailments and situations, from relieving back and neck pain to disinfecting your kitchen countertops.

Alternatives to Pharmaceuticals for Everyday Needs

If you have a cold, or are fighting bronchial symptoms or headaches, essential oils can be just as effective (or more so) as many OTC medications that address your particular symptoms. Essential oils may bring you an added benefit: They can work without all the side effects that come from many OTC pills and syrups. Some essential oils also provide disinfectant and antiviral benefits, going beyond what a pill decongestant can accomplish.

When it comes to serious illness, however, prescription pharmaceuticals, biologics, and other medications often provide the only scientifically proven means of curing disease or producing remission. In these cases, essential oils may be used in conjunction with pharmaceuticals, under a physician's guidance, to relieve discomfort, provide relaxation, and promote a sense of well-being.

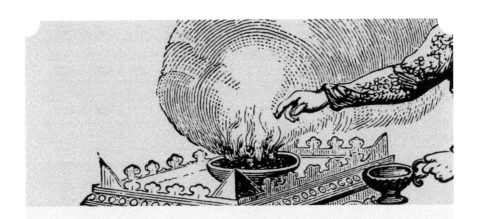

THE HEALING HAND OF GOD

And Moses said unto Aaron, Take a censer, and put fire therein from off the altar, and put on incense, and go quickly unto the congregation, and make an atonement for them: for there is wrath gone out from the Lord; the plague is begun. . . . And he stood between the dead and the living; and the plague was stayed.—Numbers 16:46–48

An uprising against Moses had begun, led by Korah, a descendant of Levi. God sent fire from heaven to consume many of Korah's followers, and then opened a crevasse in the ground to take others, but when the Israelites objected to this carnage, God sent the plague to punish them all. As the sickness swept through the congregation, Moses and Aaron saw the opportunity to save loyal Israelites by using the essences mingled in the holy incense: galbanum, myrrh, onycha, and frankincense. Aaron moved quickly to fill and ignite the incense burner, pouring the fragrant smoke out over the crowd and standing between the living and the 14,700 people who died of the plague. The plant essences saved those who were true to Moses; they were the only ones reached by the fragrant incense.

Consider the story of the man waiting for rescue on the roof of his house after a great storm had burst the levees and flooded his town. "I will trust God," the man said, "and I know he will send a divine miracle to save me." A neighbor came by in a boat and said, "Come and get into my boat, and I will take you to safety." The man shook his head and said, "No, I will wait, because God will save me."

A police motorboat came in close enough that the man could climb into the boat, but again he shook his head. "Save someone else; God will save me," he said. A rescue crew arrived in a helicopter and lowered a rope ladder to him, but again the man waved them off. "No, go help others! God will save me," he shouted to them.

Finally, the waters rose above his roof, and the man drowned. When he arrived in heaven, he stood before God and cried, "I believed in You! Why didn't You save me?" God said, "I sent you a rowboat, a motorboat, and a helicopter. What more were you expecting?"

Pharmaceuticals may not be the answer to everything, nor necessarily the first healing method we should turn to, but they are part of the vast array of miracles God provides for us on earth. When you or your loved ones face serious illness, do not turn away from these forms of rescue. These, too, are part of God's plan for health and healing.

The Science of Essential Oils

You've already learned that essential oils are the true essence of the plant and that they come from chemical compounds called terpenes (or hydrocarbons), the same molecules that create the plant's scent; every plant species has a unique combination of 100 or more terpenes that make the plant's scent different from every other plant species. These compounds also provide the plant with the ability to perform in a wide variety of ways, lending its essence to oils for medicinal uses, cleaning agents, and household and beauty products.

Essential oils differ from the oils we use in frying and sautéing, for example, because essential oils vaporize at high temperatures. The oils used in cooking are *fixed oils,* so-called because they do not change their liquid state when heated. On the following pages, you'll learn how to use olive oil and others as "carrier oils" for your essential oils.

When you inhale the fragrance of an essential oil, its volatile organic compounds remain in the olfactory membrane of your nose—the lining of your nostrils. Here, receptor neurons (nerve cells) take in the scent molecules and hold them, then send electrical impulses to your brain's olfactory bulb, the center of your sense of smell. The olfactory bulb then signals the area of your brain that contains emotional memories, while it simultaneously reaches out to your limbic system, the part of the brain that controls things such as blood pressure, heart rate, and breathing. The limbic system also controls memory and hormone balance, so once a scent reaches it, many changes can take place in your body. Fear, anger, depression, anxiety, happiness, and sadness are all regulated here. This is why aromatherapy can have such a powerful effect on the human body and its emotional state.

While there is plenty of anecdotal evidence that essential oils and aromatherapy have beneficial effects on a number of health issues, Western medical science has only begun to examine this closely. In 1999, a study conducted at the University of Buenos Aires determined that sandalwood essential oil slowed the replication of herpes simplex viruses 1 and 2 in a laboratory setting. More recently, studies have turned to the issues of antibiotic resistance in farm animals; a study published in the *Journal of Animal Science* found that rosemary and oregano essential oils killed bacteria in chickens as effectively as antibiotics. A 2016 Canadian study found that peppermint essential oil was particularly effective in keeping fruit-infesting flies off valuable crops.

You won't find much research on essential oils in the United States, for one simple reason: There isn't much money in it. Essential oils are naturally occurring substances that can't be patented, so they don't attract the interest of pharmaceutical companies looking for long-term financial gain. Plenty of scientific research on essential oils takes place overseas, however, so as we select essential oils for our use, we can still benefit from the work of scientists in Europe, Asia, and South America.

Ointment and perfume rejoice the heart.

—Proverbs 27:9

Getting Started with Essential Oils

Some books dedicate entire chapters to the selection, tools, and methods for using essential oils, but if our Biblical ancestors managed to use them with the simple tools they had available, you can master the use of essential oils with a basic kit as well. Using essential oils in your everyday life is actually an easy process, so we'll keep it simple by going over the things you need to know in a few basic steps: application methods, shopping for and using essential oils, and making your own essential oil blends.

Application Methods

With a little practice, you'll soon become comfortable with measuring, dispensing, and blending your essential oils. And, it only takes a few tries to discover the application methods that are best for you and your family.

AROMATIC APPLICATIONS

Remove the cap from a bottle of essential oil and take a whiff, and you'll get the beneficial effects immediately. This is known as *direct inhalation*—there's nothing between you and the essential oil but air. If you're looking to focus your concentration, clear your mind, battle stress, or reduce your anxiety level, this quick and effective method can help you regain control of your day. Hold the open bottle close to your nose and inhale the scent deeply several times, being careful not to inhale the oil itself into your nose (where it may be painful).

If you place a drop or two of undiluted essential oil on a cotton ball or sprinkle a little on a pillowcase, you're using *indirect inhalation*. (This is also known as using the oil *neat*.) Wipe a drop or two onto a heating vent in your home or office, or place a drop onto your car's air vents for a brief but powerful aromatic experience.

In both methods, you're using the essential oil without diluting it. Many people prefer to use a humidifier, vaporizer, or diffuser for a more penetrating and lasting effect.

- **A humidifier** keeps the air in the room moist by dispersing a fine water mist or releasing puffs of steam into the room. This can be very effective in clearing nasal passages and inducing comfortable sleep in a dry climate. Add a few drops of essential oil to the humidifier's water reservoir to relieve cold or flu symptoms, improve your mood, or sharpen your concentration.

- **A vaporizer** is a specific kind of humidifier, emitting warm steam to help clear bronchial passages and improve the air's humidity level. Some vaporizers are made to work with essential oils; the machine may have a medicine well or a heating well in which you can place your single or blended essential oils. If there's no special place to put your oils, simply add a few drops to the water in the reservoir.

- **A diffuser** is like a vaporizer, but it has no heating element; it creates a cool mist for the purpose of scenting the air. You will find literally hundreds of diffusers from which to choose, some that just create mist, and some that shut off automatically after a selected interval, shine patterns of lights to create an atmosphere of relaxation, and even play music. Choose a diffuser that is easy to clean and that runs quietly, so you can allow it to run overnight while you sleep, if you wish.

Let's be clear: You do not need one of each of these devices. No one in the Bible used a vaporizer or diffuser, though they may have added scented oil to a pot of water boiling over a fire, and used the steam to fight off an illness. It's more likely they employed direct or indirect inhalation, adding a little essential oil to their robes or scenting their bed linens, as noted in Proverbs 7:17: "I have perfumed my bed with myrrh, aloes, and cinnamon."

Many websites offer detailed descriptions of the way each mist dispenser works, so you can compare and choose the one that's best for your home or office.

Many essential oils are safe to apply to your skin when they are diluted with one or more carrier oils. Essential oils add a fragrant and therapeutic component to massage, hot compresses, cold packs, or a hot bath, and they can be added to liquid soaps, lotions, and creams to fight germs and heal dry skin.

All of these topical application methods provide dual benefits when essential oils are part of the therapeutic process. When you add an essential oil to your massage oil, for example, the oil absorbs easily into the skin, while its fragrance is released into the air as the oil warms in contact with the body. For a hot compress, add a few drops of essential oil to the water before soaking a towel in it, bringing the anti-inflammatory properties of the oil into direct skin contact while the fragrance provides calming or stimulating effects.

In chapter 4, you'll learn how to make a warm compress or a cold pack. The recipes will help you create the blends that are most effective for a wide variety of conditions and ailments.

INGESTION

In some countries, adding essential oils to food or drink is an accepted practice when done under a doctor's supervision. While many of the plants that produce essential oils also are used in seasoning and flavoring food, **ingesting the oils is not recommended**, and we discourage you from doing so. No recipes in chapter 4 contain instructions for swallowing essential oils or using them in any other invasive manner.

Shopping for Essential Oils

What is a high-quality essential oil, and how do you know if you're buying one? Many products claim to be "essential" when they are not. So, here is a primer to help you select the ones that will provide the most therapeutic benefits.

- **Bottling:** Essential oils are available only in glass bottles, because many of them will eat through plastic. If you pick up a bottle and it's plastic, chances are the oil inside is *adulterated*, meaning that it's mixed with a preservative, alcohol, or another chemical. Most essential oils must be in dark brown (amber) or blue (cobalt) glass, which keeps them from being ruined by exposure to sunlight. Essential oils in clear glass bottles may have lost some potency since they left the bottler. Keep an eye out for loose caps and dusty bottles, as well, as these may have been on the shelf for a long time. A loose cap can mean the oil has been exposed to air, so some of it may have evaporated.

- **Labeling:** If the bottle says that the oil inside is a "fragrance oil," a "nature-identical oil," a perfume, or a synthetic, it is not an essential oil. All of these terms signal that the liquid inside contains additional chemicals. That said, some essential oil bottlers use words that are equally misleading: There is no recognized standard for "pure" essential oil, so the word can mean a number of things that have nothing to do with purity. Look on the label for the oil's botanical name and method of extraction. If the oil is not steam distilled or cold pressed, it may be something other than essential.

   "Therapeutic grade" or "aromatherapy grade" are terms invented and popularized by multi-level marketing (MLM) companies that sell essential oils. These terms have no meaning within the industry, as there are no federally established grading standards in the United States. MLM companies tell customers that these claims attest to their internal standards for quality, but don't be misled into thinking that therapeutic grade somehow makes one essential oil more pure or effective than another.

- **Price:** If a brand sells all of its essential oils at the same price, you can be sure the oils are not of the highest quality. Some essential oils are more difficult to extract from plants, and some have become rare because the plants themselves are on the verge of extinction—so those oils are more expensive than others. In addition, some essential oil extractors use a process known as "bulking," in which they combine plants from the previous year's harvest with this year's fresh crop. This reduces the quality of the essential oil, which in turn reduces the price.

This is not to say that all of the most expensive essential oils are the best ones, but it's worth asking questions of your supplier before you choose which oils to purchase from whom.

- **Size:** Essential oils come in a number of different sizes. In most cases, it's best to start with a small size (most companies offer a 5-milliliter size) before investing in a larger amount, to be sure that the oil you've selected performs in the way you expect. For example, you may find that while oregano essential oil really does dissolve the skin tags you've been trying to get rid of for years, smelling like a baking pizza does not appeal to you. Some essential oils may react differently with each individual's body chemistry, as well, changing the scent in ways you don't like—or even causing a skin reaction. Perform a patch test with each oil (see page 39) before you use it liberally.

- **Starter oils:** You will find that you will use some oils immediately and often, and some only occasionally. Every person's preferences are different in terms of the scents we enjoy most, the effect the oils will have in various situations, and what we most need our oils to do. If you don't have a specific purpose in mind to start, you may want to begin with some of the most versatile and multipurpose oils: lavender, tea tree, lemon, and frankincense, for example. If you do have an ailment or several issues you're hoping to address, choose individual oils based on the recipes in chapter 4.

Some essential oil companies offer starter kits that provide a useful and versatile assortment of oils, giving you a fairly cost-effective opportunity to try out the most commonly used ones. Over time, build your personal apothecary by adding oils for disinfecting, analgesic, anti-inflammatory, fever-reducing, stress-relieving, and decongestant abilities. Soon you'll have a kit that will help you provide natural remedies for many ailments and injuries.

CHOOSING AND USING CARRIER OILS

Many essential oils need to be blended with carrier oils before they can be used topically. (Some essential oils should not be used on skin at all; check chapter 3 for warnings included in the descriptions of each essential oil found in the Bible.) Carrier oils are fixed oils; they maintain their liquid state when heated, making them good partners for essential oils that can vaporize when exposed to oxygen.

A carrier oil is used to dilute a highly concentrated essential oil, minimizing the potential that the essential oil will irritate your skin, and keeping the essential oil from disappearing before you can enjoy its benefits. Essential oil companies generally offer a line of carrier oils, but they are also available in supermarkets and natural food stores, and often for considerably lower prices.

The only carrier oil named in the Bible is olive oil. This readily available oil makes an excellent carrier for essential oils—blending easily and maintaining its consistency—but it smells like olives and that may not appeal to you. If you'd like to use something a little more conducive to cosmetic use, sweet almond oil is pleasantly fragrant and absorbs nicely into skin. Jojoba oil, hazelnut oil, and aloe vera oil are all good choices for massage, skin and hair conditioning, and applying to first-degree burns and other injuries that need tender care.

Recommended Equipment

In many cases you will need tools to combine your essential oils with carrier oils, and to store blended oils for later use. There's a wide range of paraphernalia on the market for essential oil users, but you really don't need a lot of tools at the outset. Here are the must-haves to help you get started.

- **Bottles, vials, and jars:** If you have a blend you like, mixing up a batch for later use can be a real time-saver. Have a supply of amber or cobalt bottles and jars on hand to hold your blends, and label them to help you keep track of what you have. Most of the recipes in this book will fit into a (small) 5-milliliter, 1-ounce, or 2-ounce bottle. Also, keep a few larger bottles on hand in the 8-ounce size.

- **Diffuser:** There are literally hundreds of diffuser styles on the market. Choose a fairly inexpensive one (under $20) to start, so you can begin to understand the features and determine what you like. Some require consumables, such as filter pads, however, so keep this ongoing cost in mind when you choose a diffuser.

- **Droppers and pipettes:** When possible, choose essential oils that come in bottles with an orifice reducer, a spout that allows you to dispense one drop of oil at a time. If your favorite oil doesn't come this way, have droppers of your own on hand. A glass pipette, another form of dropper, gives you better control and greatly reduces the possibility of slip-ups and waste.

- **Funnel:** When you need to transfer your blend into a bottle, a funnel is a great tool. Choose one with a small neck that fits into your bottles.

- **Atomizer:** This small pump—like the one in a perfume bottle— fits into the top of a bottle and turns the liquid into a spray mist. If you're going to spray clothing, bed linens, or the inside of your car with an oil blend, you'll need one of these.

If this all sounds like too big an investment at the start, a bag of cotton balls or a few strips of cloth can be enough to help you determine if essential oils are for you. Just add a drop of your favorite oil to a cotton ball, hold it close to your nose, inhale, and you'll begin to understand how this oil is likely to affect your mood or your health. As essential oils become a larger part of your life, you can add tools and scents as you need them.

The Safe Use of Essential Oils

"Natural" does not always mean safe, an important thing to remember when using your essential oils. The distillation or pressing processes used to extract these oils result in highly concentrated essences, which can have unintended effects when applied to skin or inhaled. Some have high hormonal content that makes them inappropriate for pregnant women or small children, and others can irritate skin. *None of these oils is safe to swallow or to place in your mouth, and they should not be inserted as suppositories.*

Before applying any essential oil directly on your skin, perform a patch test to see how your skin will react. Add 1 drop of the essential oil to 1 teaspoon of carrier oil or to a cream or wax that you know does not irritate your skin. Rub a little of this solution on the inside of your upper arm, and wait a few hours to see what happens. If redness or a rash develops, you have sensitivity to this essential oil and you should not use it in this manner.

Safe Use during Pregnancy

As you will see in chapter 3, most essential oils are not recommended for use during pregnancy. No essential oil should be used during the first trimester, and some have hormonal effects that can actually interrupt a pregnancy or encourage menstrual bleeding. Follow the warnings provided with your essential oils, and talk to your obstetrician before using any essential oil while you are pregnant.

Safe Use with Children

If you would not use an undiluted essential oil on your own skin, you most certainly should not use it on your child's skin. The absorption rate through a child's skin is much faster than it is on an adult, so the effect is faster and greater: You only need half as much oil as you would use on yourself. If an essential oil has precautions regarding use with babies and children, it will be noted in the profile precautions in chapter 3.

Safe Use with Seniors

Some studies show that certain essential oils are effective in helping senior citizens maintain memory and balance, but others can actually make medical conditions associated with the elderly even worse. Before you use any essential oil with an elderly person, check the precautions for use of that oil to be sure it will not conflict with the person's condition. If it's safe, use only half as much as you would with a younger adult. An older person's skin may become hypersensitive to some substances, so do a patch test before you apply it more broadly.

Phototoxicity

Some essential oils contain photodynamic molecules that make the skin more susceptible to the sun's ultraviolet (UV) rays. These oils react to UV light and cause sunburn. The oils themselves are not dangerous to the skin, but the way they react to UV light can be damaging—which is why this reaction is called *phototoxicity* or *photosensitivity*.

If you plan to be out in the sun, do not use the following essential oils before you do so. Note: The only Biblical oil on this list is cumin.

- Angelica
- Bergamot
- Bitter orange
- Cumin
- Dill
- Ginger
- Grapefruit
- Lemon
- Lemon verbena
- Lime
- Orange
- Tagetes
- Tangerine
- Yuzu

ESSENTIAL OILS TO AVOID

The Geneva International Fragrance Association has banned some essential oils because they are potentially carcinogenic, cause immediate skin issues, or are fatal if swallowed. Many are no longer available for consumer use. Five of the essential oils from the Bible profiled in this book are on this list. They are:

Calamus	Rue
Hyssop	Wormwood
Mustard seed	

They are explored in this book because of their inclusion in the Bible, but you must decide for yourself if you feel comfortable having these oils in your home, particularly if you have small children. None of the remedies in the book call for these oils.

In addition, these are the other essential oils that the Geneva International Fragrance Association recommends avoiding altogether:

Ajowan	Fig leaf absolute	Savin
Balsam of Peru	Horseradish	Southernwood
Bitter almond	Jaborandi	Styrax gum (Oriental sweetgum)
Boldo leaf	Massoia bark	
Cade oil crude (Prickly juniper)	Melaleuca bracteata (Black tea tree)	Tansy
		Tea absolute
Camphor	Melilotus	Thuja
Colophony (Rosin)	Ocotea	Tonka bean
Costus root (Kuth)	Parsley seed	Verbena
Croton	Santolina	Wormseed
Elecampane (scabwort)	Sassafras	

CHAPTER THREE

30 Essential Oils of the Bible

Their fruit will be for food and their leaves for healing.

—EZEKIEL 47:12

In this chapter, you will find detailed descriptions of all the essential oils that appear in the Bible. Each oil's common and botanical names are given, followed by a brief description of its use in the Bible, its scent, and its extraction method. Nearly all of the 30 oils are in common use today, with the exception of the five on the list of essential oils to avoid (see page 41), so you'll also find information on each oil's medicinal properties and uses, plus ideas for other essential oils to blend with it or use as a substitute. Every oil profile also includes any precautions about its use.

At the end of the book (see page 203), there is a catalog of the verses in Scripture in which you'll find mention of these oils. Because Scripture does not always give us a clear recipe for the way each essential oil was used, Biblical scholars have delved into the ancient history of medicine in the Middle East to find the most likely uses for each. You will find both the traditional and the modern uses for each oil in this chapter to help you find the right uses for your own home and family.

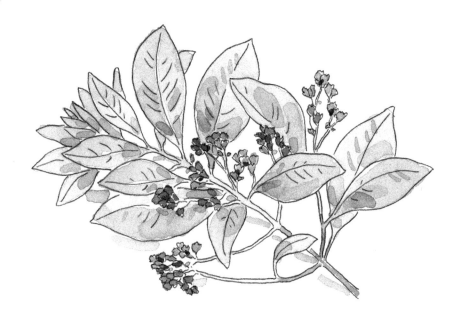

And there came also Nicodemus, which at the first came to Jesus by night, and brought a mixture of myrrh and aloes, about an hundred pound weight.

—JOHN 19:39

Aloes

Santalum album

THE ALOES USED in the Bible is not related to the aloe vera plant. Instead, the references are to the fruity, woody, warm scent of what we now call sandalwood. Aloes, along with myrrh and cassia, was part of the "oil of gladness" detailed in Psalm 45:8, and the scent appears again to perfume the seductive bed described in Proverbs 7:17. In the New Testament, aloes appears only once: Joseph of Arimathaea and Nicodemus used the fragrant aloes along with myrrh when they wrapped the body of Jesus for burial.

Many of the 16 varieties of sandalwood are now approaching extinction. This, coupled with the costly process of hydro-distillation to extract the essential oil from the heart of trees 15 years old or older, has made pure sandalwood essential oil an expensive item.

MEDICINAL PROPERTIES Analgesic, antibacterial, antiseptic, aromatic, astringent, disinfectant

MEDICINAL USES Bronchial congestion, depression, inflammation, itching, maintaining healthy skin, stress and tension, urinary tract infections

BLEND WITH Benzoin, clary sage, clove, cypress, frankincense, jasmine, myrrh, rose

SUBSTITUTE WITH Benzoin, cedarwood

PRECAUTIONS None specific

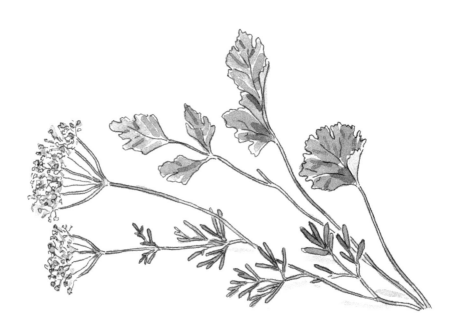

Woe unto you, scribes and Pharisees,
hypocrites! for ye pay tithe of mint and
anise and cummin, and have omitted the
weightier matters of the law, judgment,
mercy, and faith: these ought ye to have
done, and not to leave the other undone.

—MATTHEW 23:23

Anise

Pimpinella anisum

ANISE APPEARS ONLY once in the Bible, as Jesus chastises the scribes and Pharisees for paying attention to minute details of the law—represented by the tithing of tiny plants such as mint and anise—instead of the larger issues of mercy and faith. The fact that government officials of the day saw anise as something worth tithing, however, indicates its value and uses, from flavoring food to fighting infection.

The distinctly sweet, licorice scent of anise makes it an especially desirable oil for aromatherapy. Extracted from the plant's dried, ripe fruit and seeds through steam distillation, anise oil contains a potent organic compound called anethole, which has been proven to fight bacteria, yeast, and fungi. It's also effective against mosquito larvae.

MEDICINAL PROPERTIES Analgesic, antirheumatic, antiseptic, antispasmodic, decongestant, insecticidal, sedative, stimulant

MEDICINAL USES Arthritis, bronchitis, colic, cramps, epileptic episodes, flatulence, hangover, headache, indigestion, migraine, muscle pain, nasal congestion, stress, vertigo, whooping cough

BLEND WITH Caraway, cardamom, cedarwood, coriander, dill, fennel, rosewood, tangerine

SUBSTITUTE WITH Fennel, star anise

PRECAUTIONS Do not use if you are pregnant. Do not use on skin. Use sparingly.

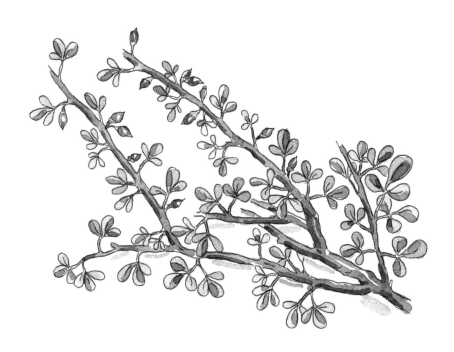

Is there no balm in Gilead; is there no physician there? Why then is not the health of the daughter of my people recovered?

—JEREMIAH 8:22

Balm

Commiphora opobalsamum, Populus balsamifera

MANY BIBLICAL SCHOLARS agree that the "balm" in the Old Testament, including the balm of Mecca and the balsam poplar, is actually the resin of one or more species of balsam tree. It's possible that the references to balm in Genesis, Jeremiah, and Ezekiel refer to two or three different plants, all of which draw their healing power from the trees' sap. Once extracted, the sap hardened into a resinous gum, to which users in Biblical times added spices and oils to apply the balm directly to the skin.

Today, balsam poplar essential oil (*Populus balsamifera*) is steam distilled from the native North American tree's buds and stems, and is the closest and most affordable analog to the balm of Gilead. Its fresh, resinous, woody scent can be a pleasant alternative to commercial topical analgesics.

MEDICINAL PROPERTIES Analgesic, anesthetic, antifungal, anti-inflammatory, antispasmodic

MEDICINAL USES Bruises, chest rub for colds and flu, muscle pain, wound care

BLEND WITH Frankincense, German chamomile, helichrysum, myrrh

SUBSTITUTE WITH German chamomile, myrrh

PRECAUTIONS People on medication metabolized by the enzyme CYP2D6 should avoid use of this oil. Check with your pharmacist before using.

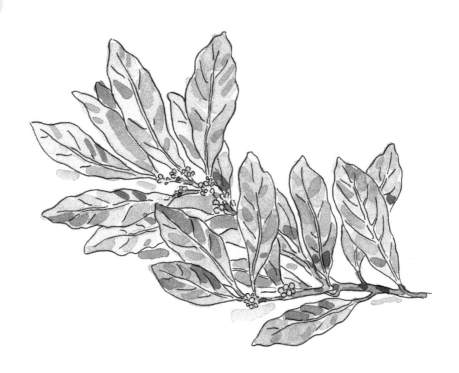

I have seen the wicked in great
power, and spreading himself
like a green bay tree.

—Psalm 37:35

Bay

Laurus nobilis

BAY APPEARS ONLY once in the Bible, in a Psalm for David—one that speaks of the ways God will care for those who believe in Him. Psalm 37 tells us that the wicked can grow strong and spread their influence far and wide, but they cannot prevail against those who believe in God's word.

Of the many varieties of bay essential oil, the spicy-sweet bay laurel, now produced by steam distillation of its leaves, is the one that was available to people of Biblical times. This evergreen tree originated in Asia, but began to appear in the Mediterranean countries well before the time of Christ. It had become quite common in the Middle East by the time it was mentioned in Psalm 37.

MEDICINAL PROPERTIES Analgesic, antibiotic, antiseptic, antispasmodic, astringent, emmenagogue, febrifuge, insecticide, sedative, sudorific

MEDICINAL USES Arthritis, circulation, colds and flu, diarrhea, hair loss prevention, muscle pain, neuralgia, skin infection

BLEND WITH Cedarwood, coriander, eucalyptus, lavender, lemon, rose, rosemary, ylang-ylang

SUBSTITUTE WITH California bay laurel, eucalyptus

PRECAUTIONS Do not use if you are pregnant. Do not use on children or for aromatherapy with children. May cause irritation to the mucous membranes and the skin. May be carcinogenic. Do not substitute mountain laurel (*Kalmia latifolia*), as this is poisonous.

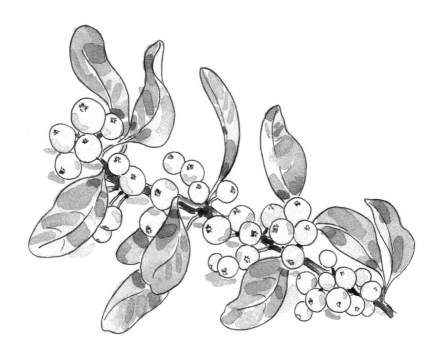

And the manna was as coriander
seed, and the colour thereof as
the colour of bdellium.

—NUMBERS 11:7

Bdellium

Commiphora wightii, Commiphora africana

THE APPEARANCE OF bdellium in the Bible seems almost deliberately confusing. Genesis relates it to onyx—thereby implying that it may be a mineral—and Numbers compares its color to the manna eaten in the desert by the followers of Moses, without providing any further explanation. However, in the ages since the five books of Moses were written, two plants valued by perfumers have produced a myrrh-like substance called bdellium or bdellion (or bedolach in Hebrew).

Today bdellium is available primarily from India under the name "guggul," in the form of an earthy, pungent resin with a hint of vanilla, or (rarely) as a steam-distilled essential oil. You can use the resin as incense or add it to your favorite carrier oil.

MEDICINAL PROPERTIES Analgesic, antiseptic, antispasmodic, astringent, relaxant, stimulant

MEDICINAL USES Bronchial disorders, menstrual cramps, throat infections, wound care

BLEND WITH Cassia, cinnamon, frankincense, galbanum, myrrh, onycha, spikenard

SUBSTITUTE WITH Myrrh

PRECAUTIONS Do not use if you are pregnant or breast-feeding. Do not use if you have a hormone-sensitive condition including endometriosis or breast, uterine, or ovarian cancer. May interfere with treatment of thyroid conditions. May stimulate bleeding, so stop using at least two weeks before scheduled surgery.

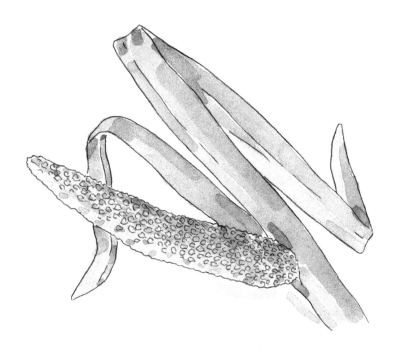

Take thou also unto thee principal spices, of pure myrrh five hundred shekels, and of sweet cinnamon half so much, even two hundred and fifty shekels, and of sweet calamus two hundred and fifty shekels.

—Exodus 30:23

Calamus

Acorus calamus

CALAMUS IS ONE of the ingredients that God specifies in His instructions to Moses for making holy anointing oil—the oil used to anoint the tabernacle and the "ark of the testimony," in the language of the King James Bible. Highly prized and revered by the people of Israel, it appears again in Song of Solomon as one of the mingled scents of the writer's dearest love and in Ezekiel as one of the many riches God bestowed upon Tyrus in the time before its predicted ruin.

Calamus—also known as sweet flag—is valued for its sweet, woodsy scent, one that calms the soul when diffused in small amounts. It is extracted from the plant's root by steam distillation.

MEDICINAL PROPERTIES
Anti-arthritic, antibiotic, antispasmodic, circulatory, stimulant, tranquilizer

MEDICINAL USES Anxiety and panic, clarity, headache, memory stimulation, muscle pain and stiffness, tension

BLEND WITH Cedarwood, cinnamon, clary sage, lavender, patchouli, rosemary, tea tree, ylang-ylang

SUBSTITUTE WITH Cinnamon, ginger, jasmine, myrrh, sandalwood

PRECAUTIONS Identified in this book as an essential oil to avoid. Do not use if you are pregnant. Do not use neat or internally, as it may cause convulsions and hallucinations. Calamus is considered carcinogenic when used in high doses. Not safe for children under 6.

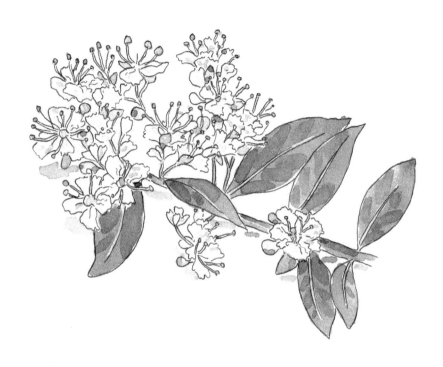

My beloved is unto me as a cluster of
camphire in the vineyards of Engedi.

—SONG OF SOLOMON 1:14

Camphire

Lawsonia inermis

CAMPHIRE—NOT TO BE confused with camphor, which is something else entirely—appears only twice in the Bible: both times in Song of Solomon's "Song of Songs," as the writer swears fidelity to an adored lover. When taken literally, this Old Testament book tells the story of King Solomon's pending marriage to Pharaoh's daughter—who, we find out later in 1 Kings, becomes an instrument in Solomon's downfall. Christians, however, see this book as an allegory for Christ as the beloved bridegroom or bride, who unites all people of the earth in their love for Him.

Today we know camphire as henna (or mehndi), a sweet oil with notes of licorice and orange, used in Egyptian and other cultures to stain fingernails red and to paint lasting (but not permanent) artwork on the body. Camphire is an absolute, derived via solvent extraction.

MEDICINAL PROPERTIES
Antibacterial, antitumor, emmenagogue, relaxant, stimulant

MEDICINAL USES Hair growth, menstrual regularity and cramps, sunscreen

BLEND WITH Lavender, neroli, Roman chamomile, rose, sandalwood, ylang-ylang

SUBSTITUTE WITH Myrtle, Roman chamomile, tea tree

PRECAUTIONS Do not use if you are pregnant. Not for use by children under 14.

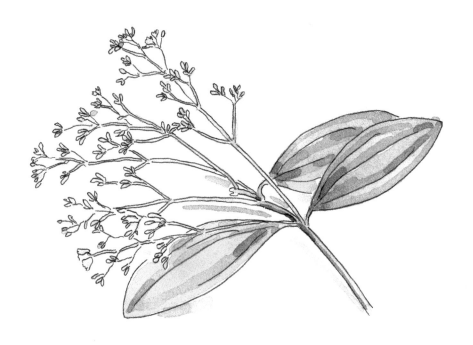

All your garments are scented
with myrrh and aloes and cassia,
out of the ivory palaces, by which
they have made you glad.

—PSALM 45:8

Cassia

Cinnamomum cassia

HOT, SPICY-SWEET CASSIA is one of the ingredients God gives Moses in Exodus when He dictates the recipe for the holy anointing oil Moses will use for the tabernacle and the Ark of the Covenant. Cited in two other Old Testament verses, cassia clearly had special value for the children of Israel, as it figures in the riches of Tyrus. In Psalms, the writer goes so far as to state that God's own garments are scented with cassia, along with myrrh and aloes.

The essential oil is steam distilled from the plant's leaves and twigs, though some products that contain cassia extract the oil from the tree's bark.

MEDICINAL PROPERTIES
Antibacterial, antigalacto-gogue, antimicrobial, antiviral, astringent, circulatory, emmenagogue, febrifuge, stimulant

MEDICINAL USES Alertness, arthritis pain, circulation, diarrhea, flatulence, menstrual cramps, mood elevation, nausea

BLEND WITH Balsam, caraway, coriander, frankincense, geranium, German chamomile, ginger, Roman chamomile, rosemary

SUBSTITUTE WITH Cinnamon

PRECAUTIONS Do not use if you are pregnant or breastfeeding. Always dilute when using on skin, as the oil can sensitize and burn. Not for use with children under 2.

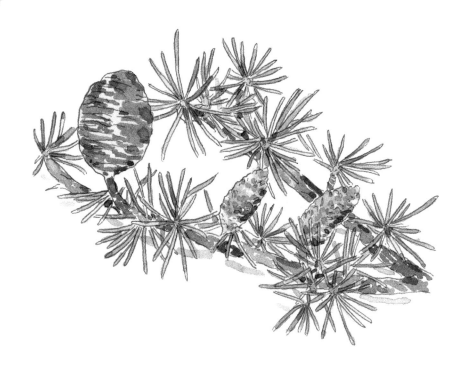

And the priest shall take cedar wood,
and hyssop, and scarlet, and cast it into
the midst of the burning of the heifer.

—NUMBERS 19:6

Cedar

Cedrus libani, Cedrus atlantica

THE CEDARS OF Lebanon, referenced 71 times in the Bible, are the ultimate symbols of towering strength and purification. In Leviticus and Numbers, cedar wood features prominently in rituals for cleansing lepers of their disease, and for cleansing priests and citizens of sin. Great kings and leaders throughout the Middle East brought cedar lumber to one another as gifts. These 90-foot-high trees were used to build their palaces and the great trunks were used to make masts for their ships. This wood was undoubtedly prized as much for its fragrance as its strength.

The cedar essential oil we use today maintains the fresh, tangy, woody scent of these majestic trees, steam distilled from the wood itself. For the closest connection to Biblical cedar, look for oils that contain species of the genus *Cedrus* rather than the ones that contain *Juniperus virginiana,* which is the North American red cedar.

MEDICINAL PROPERTIES
Antibacterial, antiseptic, antispasmodic, astringent, fungicide, insecticide, sedative

MEDICINAL USES Cystitis, dandruff, eczema, hair loss prevention, insect repellent, itching, rashes, stimulant

BLEND WITH Benzoin, cinnamon, cypress, frankincense, juniper, lavender, neroli, rose

SUBSTITUTE WITH Sandalwood

PRECAUTIONS Do not use if you are pregnant.

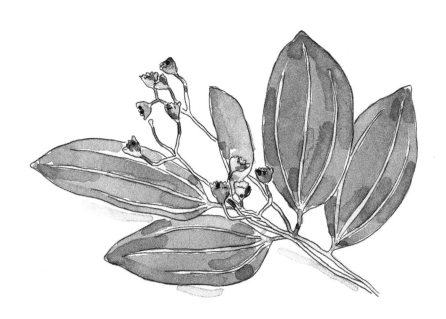

And cinnamon, and odours, and
ointments, and frankincense, and wine,
and oil, and fine flour, and wheat,
and beasts, and sheep, and horses, and
chariots, and slaves, and souls of men.

—REVELATION 18:13

Cinnamon

Cinnamomum zeylanicum

VALUED AS ONE of the ingredients of the holy anointing oil God specified to Moses, cinnamon is also listed in Revelation as one of the many forms of highly prized merchandise men will no longer desire when Babylon falls.

Today, the sweet, spicy scent we associate with cookies, curries, and other dishes also provides a number of health benefits that make it one of the most popular essential oils. Be sure to choose cinnamon essential oil steam distilled from the leaves of the tree—oils taken from the bark can be harmful to skin, and do not bring the same benefits in aromatherapy.

MEDICINAL PROPERTIES Analgesic, antibacterial, antifungal, anti-inflammatory, antiseptic, antiviral, blood sugar control, circulatory, digestive

MEDICINAL USES Acne, colds and flu, healing, indigestion, lactation, mental sharpness, menstrual bleeding and pain relief, topical infection

BLEND WITH Cardamom, geranium, lavender, lemon, orange, rosemary

SUBSTITUTE WITH Cassia

PRECAUTIONS Do not use if you are pregnant. Do not use if you take blood thinners or have hemophilia, kidney or liver disease, or prostate cancer. May cause skin irritation. Do not use with children under 6.

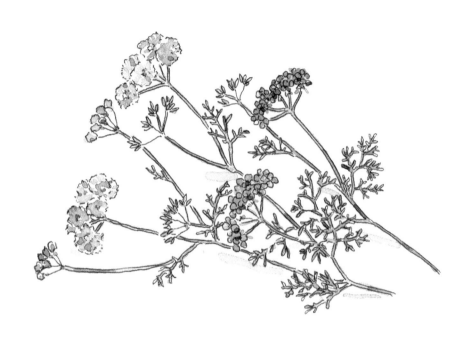

And the house of Israel called the
name thereof Manna: and it was like
coriander seed, white; and the taste of
it was like wafers made with honey.

—EXODUS 16:31

Coriander

Coriandrum sativum

CORIANDER SEED APPEARS just twice in the Bible, but both references are in descriptions of the manna that falls from heaven as Moses and the Jews wander in the desert. The manna, a gift from God to help His people survive after their rapid departure from Egypt, resembles coriander seed in its light color. Exodus tells us that its sweet taste brought joy to a people who, moments before, had believed they would perish after all, even though God had led them out of their misery as slaves to Pharaoh.

Steam distilled from coriander seed, this woody, spicy oil finishes with a lightly fruity note.

MEDICINAL PROPERTIES Analgesic, antispasmodic, aphrodisiac, deodorant, digestive, fungicide, stimulant

MEDICINAL USES Bloating, body odor, cramps, flatulence, fungal infections, pain relief, sexual desire, stimulant

BLEND WITH Bergamot, cinnamon, ginger, grapefruit, neroli, orange

SUBSTITUTE WITH Bergamot, cilantro, oregano

PRECAUTIONS None specific.

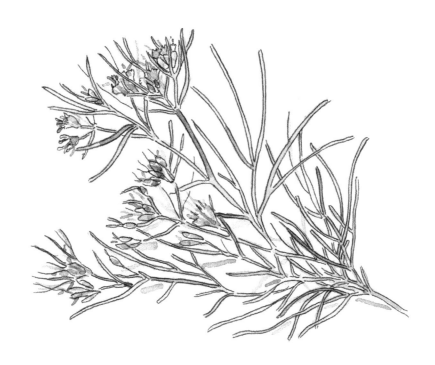

When he hath made plain the face thereof,
doth he not cast abroad the fitches,
and scatter the cumin, and cast in
the principal wheat and the appointed
barley and the rie in their place?

—ISAIAH 28:25

Cumin

Cuminum cyminum

WELL KNOWN IN ancient Egypt as both a spice and a preservative, particularly in mummification, cumin (or "cummin" in the King James Version of the Bible) is one of the three plants specifically called out by Jesus in his chastisement of the Pharisees. He uses cumin, anise, and mint as an analogy for the minute points of law these officials examined, instead of the greater issues of judgment and mercy that would refocus Jewish law to benefit its people. Thousands of years earlier, in Isaiah, cumin was used as a metaphor for one of the responsibilities of daily life God instructs His people to carry out properly in His name.

Cumin essential oil is steam distilled from the plant's seeds, producing a warm, nutty scent with the thrill of spicy heat.

MEDICINAL PROPERTIES Antibacterial, antiseptic, antispasmodic, diuretic, emmenagogue, stimulant

MEDICINAL USES Aging skin, anxiety, flatulence, menstrual issues, post-menopause symptoms, stress, topical infection

BLEND WITH Angelica, caraway, coriander, Roman chamomile

SUBSTITUTE WITH Caraway, coriander

PRECAUTIONS Do not use if you are pregnant. It is photosensitizing: Do not apply it to skin before going out in the sun. Large amounts can cause headaches and nausea.

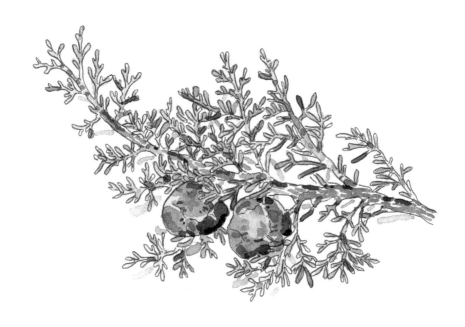

He heweth him down cedars, and
taketh the cypress and the oak, which
he strengtheneth for himself among
the trees of the forest: he planteth an
ash, and the rain doth nourish it.

—ISAIAH 44:14

Cypress

Cupressus sempervirens

CYPRESS APPEARS ONLY once in the Bible, as God describes to Isaiah the fate of the smith and the carpenter who make graven images in direct defiance of God's commandments. Cypress, along with oak and cedar, is a strong, useful material God provides for man's use in building fires for warmth, baking, and cooking. Later in the chapter, however, He warns that some men use the ashes, or "residue" of such fire, to fashion idols for worship—and no good will come to them for this.

We can infer from this chapter of Isaiah that using the clean, fresh scent of cypress essential oil in your home obeys God's word in the literal sense. Be sure to choose the pure essential oil that has been steam distilled from the tree's branches.

MEDICINAL PROPERTIES Antiseptic, antispasmodic, astringent, deodorant, respiratory, sedative, sudorific

MEDICINAL USES Bleeding control, body odor, hair loss prevention, promotion of sweating, respiratory care, skin and muscle tightening, spasms, wound care

BLEND WITH Bergamot, citrus, clary sage, frankincense, juniper, lavender, pine, sandalwood

SUBSTITUTE WITH Arborvitae, fir, juniper, wintergreen

PRECAUTIONS Do not use if you are pregnant.

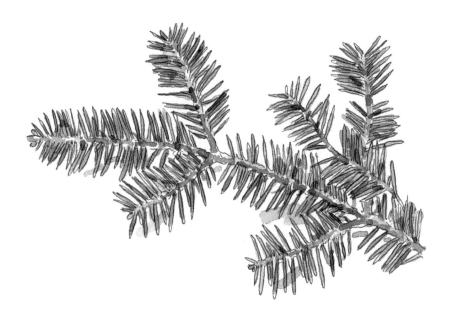

I will plant in the wilderness the cedar,
the shittah tree, and the myrtle, and the oil tree;
I will set in the desert the fir tree, and the
pine, and the box tree together: That they may
see, and know, and consider, and understand
together, that the hand of the Lord hath done
this, and the Holy One of Israel hath created it.

—ISAIAH 41:19–20

Fir

Abies balsamea

FIR APPEARS OFTEN in the Old Testament as a building material or as a naturally occurring figure of strength that men should emulate. Musical instruments are made of it, kings exchange fir trees for great stores of food, and King Solomon orders that his "great house" be built of it. The Bible even goes so far as to give the fir tree human characteristics, as in Isaiah 14:8, "Yea, the fir trees rejoice at thee," and in Zechariah 11:2, "Howl, fir tree; for the cedar is fallen." Clearly these trees played multiple roles in the lives of kings, prophets, and common people, offering strength and shelter as well as medicinal benefits.

Of the fir essential oils you will find online and in catalogs—all steam distilled from the needles—the woodsy-fresh balsam fir (*Abies balsamea*) is the most closely associated with the oil of Biblical times. Silver, white, and Douglas fir essential oils all offer similar scents and medicinal properties, if the more common balsam fir oil is not at hand.

MEDICINAL PROPERTIES Analgesic, anti-inflammatory, antiviral, decongestant

MEDICINAL USES Arthritis, bronchitis, chronic sinus issues, colds and flu, cough, muscle pain

BLEND WITH Benzoin, lavender, lemon, orange, pine, rosemary

SUBSTITUTE WITH Cinnamon, helichrysum, myrrh, patchouli, spearmint

PRECAUTIONS May cause skin irritation.

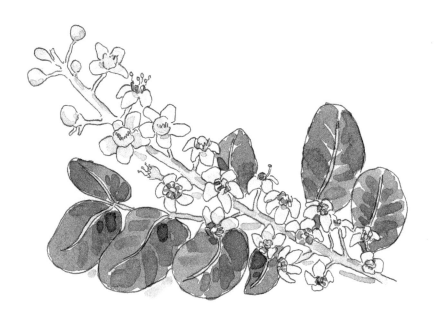

And when they were come into the house,
they saw the young child with Mary his
mother, and fell down, and worshipped
him: and when they had opened their
treasures, they presented unto him gifts;
gold, and frankincense, and myrrh.

—MATTHEW 2:11

Frankincense

Boswellia sacra, B. frereana, B. papyrifera, B. serrata

GOLD, FRANKINCENSE, AND myrrh, the offerings brought by the wise men to the newborn Jesus, are perhaps the most famous gifts ever given. This reference may have been the first time most people heard of these highly prized spices, but frankincense actually was in use from the early days of the Old Testament, prescribed by God to Moses as part of the holy anointing oil used on the Ark of the Covenant and in the sacred temple.

Today's "frank" comes from the sap of a number of trees, collected by hand-tapping the trunks to gather the piney, citrusy-scented resin for fractional distillation. In Jewish rituals, frankincense is known by its Hebrew name, olibanum.

MEDICINAL PROPERTIES Analgesic, anti-inflammatory, antiseptic, digestive, disinfectant, diuretic, sedative

MEDICINAL USES Anxiety and stress, bloating, hair and skin care, improve breathing (anti-asthma), swelling and inflammation

BLEND WITH Citrus, cypress, geranium, rose, sandalwood, ylang-ylang

SUBSTITUTE WITH Cedarwood, sandalwood

PRECAUTIONS None specific

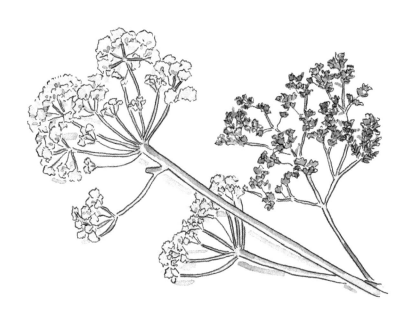

And the Lord said unto Moses, Take unto thee sweet spices, stacte, and onycha, and galbanum; these sweet spices with pure frankincense: of each shall there be a like weight.

—EXODUS 30:34

Galbanum

Ferula gummosa, F. galbaniflua

IN EXODUS, GOD calls on Moses to mix a specific set of spices into sweet-smelling incense, known in the Jewish religion as Ketoret, which is then used to consecrate the tabernacle that will house the Ten Commandments. As this is the only mention of this aromatic resin in the Bible, galbanum has had special connotation throughout history, not only to Jews but also to Christians, who saw its bitterness among the sweet as a reminder of the effects of sin.

Today's steam distillation of the gum banishes this dark note, yielding a green, floral scent with a touch of malt.

MEDICINAL PROPERTIES
Antispasmodic, circulatory, decongestant, diuretic, emmenagogue, insecticide, sedative

MEDICINAL USES Acne scars, aging skin, arthritis and other inflammation, cough, head lice, insect bites, muscle spasms, skin disorders and wound care

BLEND WITH Benzoin, fir, geranium, ginger, lavender, pine

SUBSTITUTE WITH Cedarwood

PRECAUTIONS If using with benzoin, watch for cross-sensitization, which could be present as redness, itching, or an eczema-like patch.

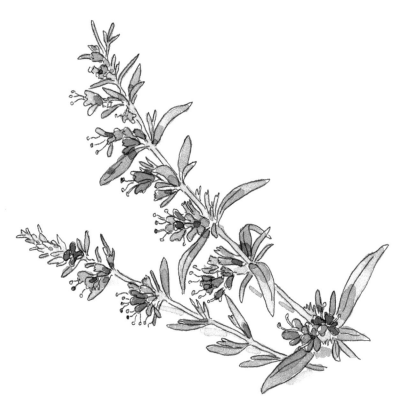

Now there was set a vessel full of vinegar:
and they filled a spunge with vinegar, and
put it upon hyssop, and put it to his mouth.

—JOHN 19:29

Hyssop

Hyssopus officinalis

THE BIBLE CONTAINS a number of references to hyssop, but the most poignant is the use of a hyssop branch (presumably) to lift the vinegar-soaked sponge to the lips of Jesus moments before his death on the cross. God also commands Moses to use hyssop to spread the blood of a bird through a house to cleanse it of leprosy. "Purge me with hyssop, and I shall be clean," Psalm 51 tells us, a further assurance that the use of this plant brings detoxification to mind and home.

Today, hyssop is produced through steam distillation and gives off a mild scent.

MEDICINAL PROPERTIES Antiseptic, antispasmodic, astringent, expectorant, febrifuge, stimulant, sudorific

MEDICINAL USES Aging skin, colds and flu, cough, cuts and scars, menstrual symptoms, promotion of perspiration, wound care

BLEND WITH Bay, geranium, myrtle, orange, rosemary, sage

SUBSTITUTE WITH Cedarwood, fir, galbanum

PRECAUTIONS Identified in this book as an essential oil to avoid. Do not use with small children. Those diagnosed with epilepsy should avoid this oil, as it can cause seizures.

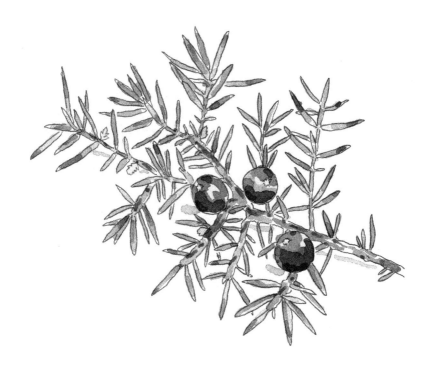

But he himself went a day's journey into the wilderness, and came and sat down under a juniper tree: and he requested for himself that he might die; and said, It is enough; now, O Lord, take away my life; for I am not better than my fathers. And as he lay and slept under a juniper tree, behold, then an angel touched him and said unto him, Arise and eat.

—1 KINGS 19:4–5

Juniper

Juniperus communis

WHEN ELIJAH SLAYS the prophets who worshipped the false god Baal, he travels a day's journey into the wilderness, sits alone under a juniper tree, and asks the Lord to take away his life. Instead, God sends an angel with a cake and water, and bids Elijah "arise and eat."

Juniper continues today as a symbol of strength and endurance, its tangy wood fragrance a source of calm, and its oil—steam distilled from the needles, wood, and berries—an antiseptic with proven healing capability.

MEDICINAL PROPERTIES
Analgesic, anti-inflammatory, antimicrobial, antiseptic, diuretic, insecticide, sedative

MEDICINAL USES Acne, anxiety, arthritis, cellulite, eczema, fatigue, gout, hangover, insect repellent, menstrual symptoms, muscle pain, nervousness, prostatitis, psoriasis, skin care, stress, wound care

BLEND WITH Bay, cedarwood, citrus, cypress, ginger, lavender, myrrh, peppermint, spikenard, tea tree

SUBSTITUTE WITH Cypress, fir

PRECAUTIONS Do not use if you are pregnant. May cause skin irritation. Do not use if you have kidney or liver disease. Not safe for children under 6.

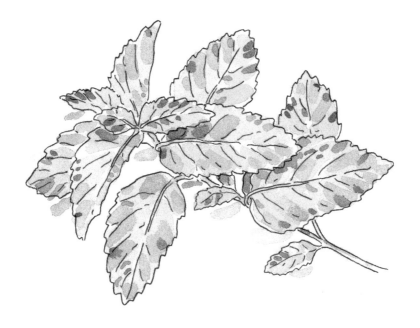

Woe to you, scribes and Pharisees, hypocrites! For you pay tithe of mint and anise and cummin, and have neglected the weightier matters of the law: justice and mercy and faith. These you ought to have done, without leaving the others undone.

—MATTHEW 23:23

Mint

Mentha spicata, Mentha longifolia

ALONG WITH ANISE and cumin, mint is one of the three plants specifically mentioned by Jesus as he argues with the Pharisees—leaders of the Jewish school of thought that became the basis for modern orthodox Judaism—about their focus on the literal interpretation of the law instead of the greater good. Mint had enough significance and value to require tithing, so the herb itself likely served people well as a cleaning aid, deodorant, and curative.

Of the list of steam-distilled essential oils in the *Mentha* family, only spearmint (*Mentha spicata*) and horse mint (*Mentha longifolia*) grew in abundance in the Middle East in Biblical times. Spearmint essential oil is milder than peppermint and is safer for use with children; horse mint is more unusual in essential oil home apothecaries.

MEDICINAL PROPERTIES Analgesic, anesthetic, antibacterial, anti-inflammatory, antiseptic, antispasmodic, decongestant, diuretic, expectorant

MEDICINAL USES Acne, air freshener, asthma, bronchitis, clarity, cold, colic, cough, fever, flatulence, headache, hiccups, laryngitis, migraine, muscle pain, nausea

BLEND WITH Basil, benzoin, eucalyptus, jasmine, lavender, lemon, peppermint, rosemary

SUBSTITUTE WITH Peppermint

PRECAUTIONS Avoid use with homeopathic remedies. If using horse mint, avoid contact with eyes, and do not use with children under 6.

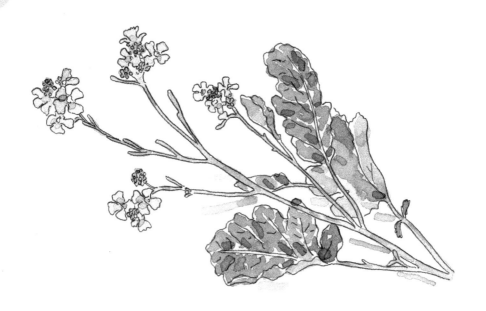

Another parable put he forth unto them,
saying, The kingdom of heaven is like to
a grain of mustard seed, which a man
took, and sowed in his field: Which indeed
is the least of all seeds: but when it is
grown, it is the greatest among herbs, and
becometh a tree, so that the birds of the air
come and lodge in the branches thereof.

—MATTHEW 13:31–32

Mustard Seed

Brassica nigra, B. juncea

IN THE PARABLE in Matthew 13:31 (repeated in Luke 13), Jesus uses the tiny mustard seed as a metaphor for the coming strength of his church. When sowed by one man, the mustard seed grows to be "the greatest among herbs," just as the church of Jesus Christ will one day become great and fill the world with righteousness. It also will attract the birds—an analogy to those from outside the immediate faith, who will be attracted to the tree of life (Jesus) as it expands.

Mustard seed essential oil, steam distilled from crushed, fermented seeds, provides a hot, eye-watering aroma reminiscent of horseradish.

MEDICINAL PROPERTIES Analgesic, antibacterial, antifungal, anti-inflammatory, decongestant, irritant, stimulant

MEDICINAL USES Arthritis, blood circulation, colds, cough, fungal infection, hair revitalizer, headache, insect repellent, promotion of sweating, returns feeling to numbed extremities

BLEND WITH Because of its strong eye-watering effects, mustard seed essential oil is not used in blends.

SUBSTITUTE WITH None

PRECAUTIONS Identified in this book as an essential oil to avoid. Not recommended for aromatherapy. Do not use on rashes or if you are prone to skin allergies. Keep away from eyes.

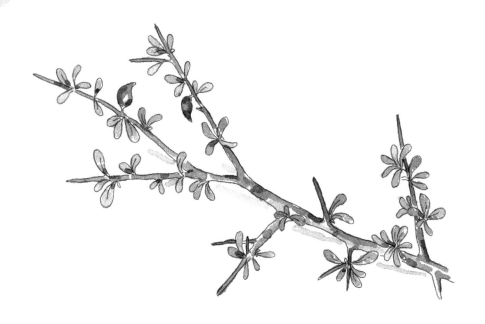

And Nicodemus, who at first came to Jesus by night, also came, bringing a mixture of myrrh and aloes, about a hundred pounds. Then they took the body of Jesus, and bound it in strips of linen with the spices, as the custom of the Jews is to bury. Now in the place where He was crucified there was a garden, and in the garden a new tomb in which no one had yet been laid.

—JOHN 19:39–41

Myrrh

Commiphora myrrha

MYRRH HAD ALREADY developed a reputation as one of the most versatile and highly prized spices in the Biblical era long before the Magi brought it as a gift to the baby Jesus. Indeed, in Genesis, Jacob's sons bring it as one of their gifts to the vizier of Egypt—whom they did not know was their brother, Joseph—and women, including Esther, use it as part of their purification rituals. In God's specifications for the holy anointing oil Moses would mix for the sacred temple, myrrh is the first and most abundant in the list. The Psalms and the Song of Solomon sing praises to myrrh's unique scent. Finally, Joseph and Nicodemus use the spice mixed with aloes to bind with cloth around the body of Jesus after his crucifixion.

Steam distilled from its resin, myrrh serves well as an aid to meditation, a key ingredient in skin balms and—most popularly—in scented candles and potpourri in your home as Christmas draws near.

MEDICINAL PROPERTIES
Antifungal, anti-inflammatory, antimicrobial, antiseptic, antiviral, expectorant, fungicide, sedative

MEDICINAL USES Aging skin, athlete's foot, bronchitis, dental health, diarrhea, dysentery, halitosis, hemorrhoids, meditation, muscle pain, ringworm, skin care, stretch marks, wound care

BLEND WITH Benzoin, citrus oils, clove, cypress, frankincense, geranium, juniper, lavender, sandalwood, spikenard

SUBSTITUTE WITH Fir, frankincense, helichrysum

PRECAUTIONS Do not use if you are pregnant or breastfeeding.

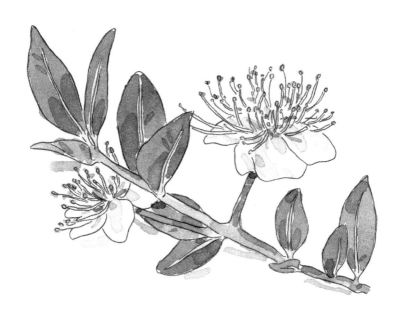

Instead of the thorn shall come up the fir tree, and instead of the brier shall come up the myrtle tree: and it shall be to the Lord for a name, for an everlasting sign (that) shall not be cut off.

—ISAIAH 55:13

Myrtle

Myrtus communis

ONE OF THE four tree species determined to be used to build booths for the Feast of Tabernacles (the Jewish holiday of Sukkot), the myrtle tree serves throughout the Old Testament as a symbol for the strength of the Jewish people. The tree is not mentioned in the New Testament, but its importance is articulated in Scripture, in Isaiah 41:19–20 and again in Isaiah 55:13, which defines myrtle as a direct representation of God, "an everlasting sign that shall not be cut off."

Steam distillation of the leaves and twigs produces the herbaceous aroma, which is very different from the sweet scent of the tree's blooming flowers, so do not expect the luscious perfume of its white blossoms. Look for the essential oil produced from plants grown in Spain or Morocco.

MEDICINAL PROPERTIES Antiseptic, aphrodisiac, astringent, deodorant, disinfectant, expectorant, sedative

MEDICINAL USES Acne, aging skin, anxiety, body odor, colds, sexual desire, sinus and chest congestion, skin care, stress, wound care

BLEND WITH Benzoin, cedarwood, coriander, eucalyptus, frankincense, lavender, myrrh, rose, ylang-ylang

SUBSTITUTE WITH Camphor, fir, helichrysum, myrrh, spearmint

PRECAUTIONS None specific

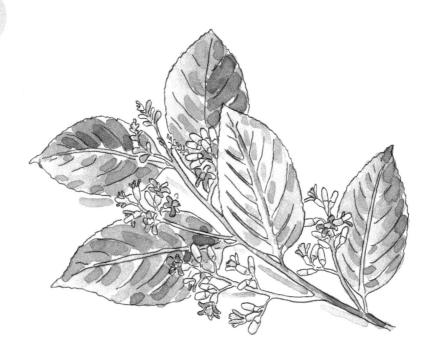

And the Lord said unto Moses, Take
unto thee sweet spices, stacte, and
onycha, and galbanum; these sweet
spices with pure frankincense: of
each shall there be a like weight.

—Exodus 30:34

Onycha

Styrax benzoin

BIBLICAL SCHOLARS DIFFER in their definitions of onycha, referred to in Scripture as a "sweet spice"—one of three spices used in the incense Moses produces in accordance with God's specific instructions. It's most likely that onycha is a plant resin that shines like the shellfish from which it takes its Latin name. The resin comes from the benzoin tree, so most essential oil bottlers call it benzoin. As the benzoin tree now grows only in Java, Sumatra, and Malaysia, the essential oil you can purchase today does not have an origin in the Biblical region. (This benzoin is not related to the organic chemical compound benzoin, but rather to benzoic acid, a naturally occurring substance in many plants.)

To extract the oil, companies use solvents that are removed once they obtain the oil. Benzoin has a distinct vanilla scent, and is most often used as "tincture of benzoin," created by adding the oil to alcohol.

MEDICINAL PROPERTIES Antidepressant, anti-inflammatory, antirheumatic, antiseptic, astringent, deodorant, disinfectant, relaxant, sedative

MEDICINAL USES Anxiety, arthritis, body odor, bronchitis, chest and nasal congestion, dry skin, flatulence, household disinfectant, inflammation, mood elevation, skin tone, tension, wound care

BLEND WITH Citrus oils, coriander, frankincense, juniper, lavender, myrrh, rose, sandalwood

SUBSTITUTE WITH Cedarwood, sandalwood

PRECAUTIONS Excessive inhalation can cause headaches, nausea, and vomiting. May cause skin sensitivity.

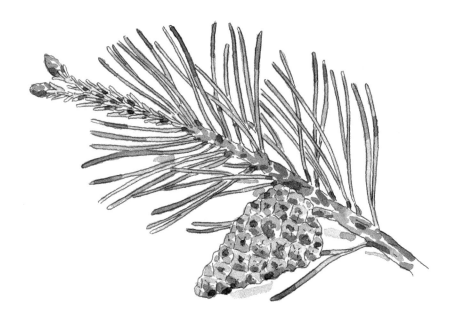

The glory of Lebanon shall come unto thee, the fir tree, the pine tree, and the box together, to beautify the place of my sanctuary; and I will make the place of my feet glorious.

—ISAIAH 60:13

Pine

Pinus

ONE OF THE trees in Isaiah's list of "the glory of Lebanon," pine also appears in God's instructions for building *sukkah,* the booths constructed for the Feast of Tabernacles. God promises, in Isaiah, that He will plant pine trees in the desert to provide for the people of Israel, especially the poor and needy.

Most pine essential oil comes from *Pinus sylvestris,* the Scotch pine—despite recent scientific evidence that this tree yields the smallest amount of essential oil of a wide range of pine trees tested. This tall, fragrant tree is a cousin to *Pinus pinea* and *Pinus brutia,* the pine species that grow in Lebanon. Essential oil from the two Middle Eastern pine species is hard to find, however, and the readily available Scotch pine provides largely the same benefits as the pines of Lebanon. The fresh, woody, tangy oil is steam distilled from the tree's needles.

MEDICINAL PROPERTIES
Analgesic, antibacterial, anti-inflammatory, antiseptic, disinfectant, expectorant, stimulant

MEDICINAL USES Acne, anxiety, athlete's foot, chest congestion, cleaning, colds and flu, dandruff, eczema, itching, mood elevation, muscle aches and pains, redness and swelling, respiratory infections, urinary tract infections

BLEND WITH Bay, cedarwood, clary sage, cypress, eucalyptus, fir, frankincense, juniper, myrrh, sandalwood, spikenard, tea tree

SUBSTITUTE WITH Cedarwood, eucalyptus, fir, myrtle, rosemary, spruce

PRECAUTIONS May cause irritation of skin and mucous membranes.

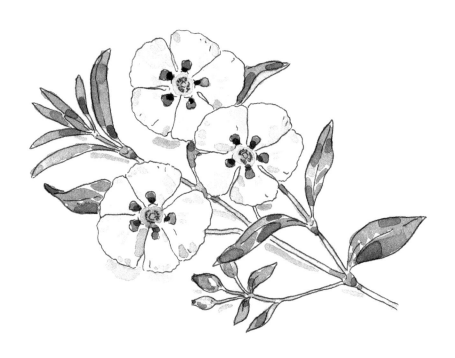

I am the rose of Sharon, and
the lily of the valleys.

—SONG OF SOLOMON 2:1

Rose of Sharon

Cistus ladaniferus, Cistus ladanifer

SHARON IS BELIEVED to be the plain between the mountains of central Palestine and the Mediterranean Sea, an area where verdant foliage probably thrived. The region's "rose"—thought actually to have been a crocus or meadow saffron—is mentioned only once in the Bible, and then poetically rather than with substance. It is clear the reference is meant as a romantic compliment to the writer's beloved. Christian scholars later interpreted this Old Testament book to be an allegory for the coming of Christ, and a prediction of the growth of Christianity that would follow. The rose of Sharon is considered a symbol of Christ himself.

The flower called rose of Sharon today—a pink bloom in the hibiscus or mallow family—is not the one the writer of Song of Solomon would have encountered. We can't be absolutely sure what flower was meant, but cistus essential oil—steam distilled from the leaves of the rock rose (also known as the labdanum) found in the Middle East—provides a close approximation with its sweet, musky scent and warm undertone.

MEDICINAL PROPERTIES
Anti-arthritic, antimicrobial, astringent

MEDICINAL USES Acne, aging skin, cramps, eczema, meditation, psoriasis, swollen lymph glands, wound care

BLEND WITH Bergamot, clary sage, cypress, helichrysum, juniper, lavender, orange, pine, Roman chamomile, sandalwood, vetiver

SUBSTITUTE WITH Galbanum, myrtle, tea tree

PRECAUTIONS Do not use if you are pregnant.

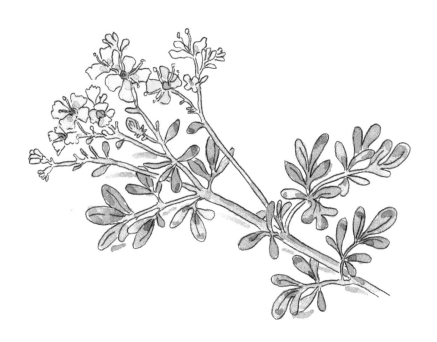

But woe unto you, Pharisees! for ye
tithe mint and rue and all manner of
herbs, and pass over judgment and the
love of God: these ought ye to have done,
and not to leave the other undone.

—LUKE 11:42

Rue

Ruta graveolens

WHILE THE GOSPEL of Matthew lists mint, anise, and cumin as the plants tithed by the Pharisees, Luke substitutes rue and "all manner of herbs." Here the reference takes into account rue's small stature—it's often used today as a border plant in gardens—as well as the use of its leaves and berries in cooking. Jesus expresses his frustration that the leaders of the Jewish people would make the tithe of a fairly unimpressive little herb a high priority instead of taking on the larger challenges of the day, but his words do not discount rue's significant place in everyday life.

Rue essential oil, steam distilled from the twigs, leaves, and berries, has a strong, bitter scent.

MEDICINAL PROPERTIES
Anti-arthritic, antibacterial, antifungal, emmenagogue, insecticide, sedative

MEDICINAL USES Airborne insect repellent, athlete's foot, botulism, epileptic seizures, disinfectant, joint pain, nervousness, salmonella, tetanus

BLEND WITH Bay, benzoin, fennel, frankincense, myrrh, thyme

SUBSTITUTE WITH Basil, cedarwood, eucalyptus

PRECAUTIONS Identified in this book as an essential oil to avoid. Do not use if you are pregnant. Keep undiluted oil away from skin and eyes.

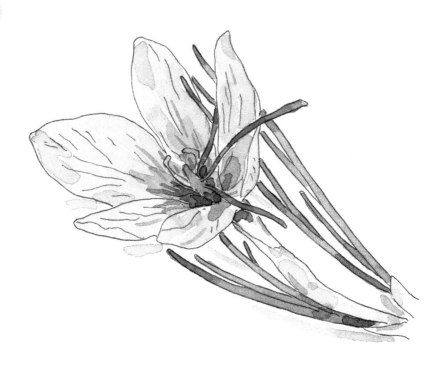

Spikenard and saffron, calamus and
cinnamon, with all trees of frankincense;
myrrh and aloes, with all the chief spices.

—SONG OF SOLOMON 4:14

Saffron

Crocus sativus

SONG OF SOLOMON reaches an exhilarating height in chapter 4, as the lover describes the spouse's every aspect in detail. Here we learn the figurative garden enclosing the spouse is filled with "pleasant fruits" and sweet-smelling herbs and spices, including saffron. Nowhere else in the Bible does saffron appear, but this one mention makes it an especially rare and costly extravagance.

Many Christian scholars believe that this entire book of the Bible refers not to King Solomon and his courtship of the daughter of Pharaoh, but to Christ himself and his spiritual presence on earth long before his birth as Jesus in the New Testament. Others see these passages as a metaphor for Israel's desire to unite with Lebanon—indeed, the chapter makes many symbolic references to military might—and to enjoy the country's protection sealed inside the "garden."

Today saffron is the most expensive spice in the world, and its essential oil ranks among the priciest as well. The yield per plant is very tiny; in fact, it takes 75,000 plants to make one pound of saffron spice. The steam-distillation process that produces the oil brings out its woody, spicy scent, with an underlying note of open grassland.

MEDICINAL PROPERTIES
Analgesic, antidepressant, anti-inflammatory, blood sugar regulation, immunity, neutralization of free radicals

MEDICINAL USES Acne, colic, cough, diabetes, flatulence, hair growth, male sexual performance, menopausal symptoms, menstrual symptoms, skin care, weight loss, wound care

BLEND WITH Rose

SUBSTITUTE WITH Cumin

PRECAUTIONS Do not use in large amounts.

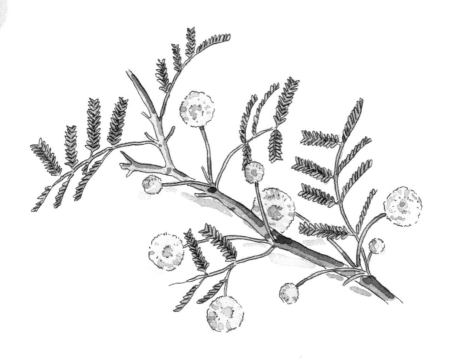

And they shall make an ark of shittim
wood: two cubits and a half shall be
the length thereof, and a cubit and
a half the breadth thereof, and a
cubit and a half the height thereof.

—EXODUS 25:10

Shittah

Acacia farnesiana

THE SHITTAH TREE figures prominently in Exodus as one of the most prominent materials for the sanctuary God orders Moses to build. Exodus provides us with a lively account of the construction of this sanctuary, detailing the generosity and devotion of the people of Israel in giving up their own possessions to make the temple and cover parts of it in gold and jewels. The shittah is a large tree that produces gum arabic, which the people of the time may have used as a binder in food, as well as to create glue and other useful substances.

Historians believe that the shittah tree is actually in the acacia family, so later translations of the Bible replace "shittah" and "shittim" (the plural of shittah) with "acacia." This lovely flowering tree produces bright yellow blossoms that yield small amounts of powdery-scented, floral essential oil through steam distillation. Even a tiny bottle of "cassie" oil will be among the most expensive essential oils you own, and it is hard to find, so you may want to use one of the substitutes for this oil's fairly narrow health benefits. You are more likely to find it as a solvent-extracted absolute.

MEDICINAL PROPERTIES
Antibacterial, probiotic

MEDICINAL USES Colds, cough, indigestion, inflammation or irritation, wound care

BLEND WITH Gardenia, honeysuckle, hyacinth, narcissus, rose

SUBSTITUTE WITH Helichrysum, lavender, Roman chamomile, tea tree

PRECAUTIONS Do not confuse cassie essential oil with cassia. Cassia essential oil is in the cinnamon family and has very different characteristics.

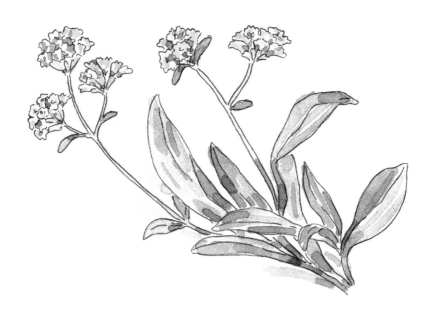

Then took Mary a pound of ointment
of spikenard, very costly, and anointed
the feet of Jesus, and wiped his feet
with her hair; and the house was
filled with the odour of the ointment.

—JOHN 12:3

Spikenard

Nardostachys jatamansi

SPIKENARD, A MEMBER of the honeysuckle family, holds a special place in Biblical history as the key ingredient in the ointment used by Mary, sister of Lazarus, to anoint the feet of Jesus. As told in John 12:4–8, she does this as an indication of her gratitude and her love for Jesus for raising her brother from the dead, yet Judas Iscariot is quick to criticize such use of the costly ointment. "Why was not this ointment sold for three hundred pence, and given to the poor?" he asks. Jesus responds just as quickly in Mary's defense: "Let her alone: against the day of my burying hath she kept this. For the poor always ye have with you; but me ye have not always."

Today we can fill our own homes with the same mossy scent. The oil is steam distilled from the plant's resin taken from the stem, and is one of the mildest and most widely beneficial of the essential oils named in the Bible.

MEDICINAL PROPERTIES
Antibacterial, antifungal, anti-inflammatory, deodorant, laxative, sedative

MEDICINAL USES Anxiety, athlete's foot, body odor, foot care, fungal infections, inflammation, mood elevation, nervous disorders, relaxation, skin care, urinary tract infections, wound care

BLEND WITH Frankincense, lavender, myrrh, orange, rose, vetiver

SUBSTITUTE WITH Cassia, lavender, tea tree

PRECAUTIONS None specified

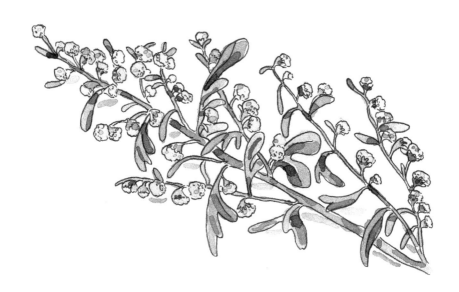

And the name of the star is called
Wormwood: and the third part of
the waters became wormwood; and
many men died of the waters,
because they were made bitter.

—REVELATION 8:11

Wormwood

Artemisia herba-alba

SCRIPTURE SPEAKS OF wormwood as bitter, noting that people died when they drank from waters tainted with it. This is the prognostication among the vivid imagery of Revelation, as the seven angels blow their trumpets one by one, and a star called Wormwood falls from heaven.

Indeed, the steam-distilled wormwood essential oil has a bitter odor. It has some specific therapeutic effects that are fairly rare among essential oils, but other remedies are equally effective and less toxic overall. Wormwood contains the chemical thujone, a neurotoxin that can cause seizures if used over a prolonged period or in significant amounts. Keep in mind that this green liquid is the basis for absinthe, an alcoholic beverage popularized in the late nineteenth and early twentieth centuries and long since banned in its true, thujone-containing form in the United States and many other countries.

MEDICINAL PROPERTIES Deodorant, digestive, emmenagogue, febrifuge, insecticide, relaxant, tonic, vermifuge

MEDICINAL USES Acid indigestion, acid reflux, body odor, fever, insect repellent, menstrual symptoms, nervous symptoms, tonic

BLEND WITH Jasmine, lavender, orange

SUBSTITUTE WITH Anise, bay, cassia, frankincense, galbanum, helichrysum

PRECAUTIONS Identified in this book as an essential oil to avoid, as it is poisonous. Can cause convulsions, restlessness, impulsive behavior, permanent brain damage, and death.

CHAPTER FOUR

Remedies and Recipes

The fruit thereof shall be for meat, and the leaf thereof for medicine.

—EZEKIEL 47:12

Now that you have a solid understanding of the essential oils in the Bible, it's time to put them to good use. You'll find many useful recipes in this chapter to help you use the natural powers of these and other essential oils in your own home. Many of these remedies include essential oils beyond those found in the Bible, so you have the opportunity to make the most of oils from all over the world, all of which are part of God's global creation.

Whether you want to open breathing passages during a cold or the flu, slow the advancement of aging skin, bring natural antibacterial agents into your kitchen, or freshen your laundry with a breath of spring, essential oils can be your go-to solution.

Acne

Thanks to medical science, we know that acne is a skin condition aggravated by hormonal changes in the body—and not a reaction to chocolate. Cleansing the skin properly helps those stricken with blemishes fight the production of sebum, the oily substance that clogs pores. Replicated studies in Australia and India have determined that tea tree essential oil is as effective at fighting acne (killing the specific bacteria that cause acne) as the pharmaceutical benzoyl peroxide, so you can battle a breakout with a natural, cost-effective remedy.

NEAT ACNE SWAB

Makes 1 treatment

2 drops tea tree essential oil

1. In the morning, wash your face with mild soap and water, and dry with a clean towel.
2. Place 2 drops of tea tree essential oil on a cotton swab or cotton ball.
3. Gently dab each pimple with the cotton swab or ball.

ACNE NIGHT TREATMENT

Makes 10 treatments

30 drops orange essential oil
15 drops carrot seed essential oil
5 drops juniper essential oil
5 drops Roman chamomile essential oil

1. In a small glass or metal bowl, mix the orange, carrot seed, juniper, and Roman chamomile essential oils neat (undiluted), and pour the mixture into a small (5-mL) dark amber or cobalt glass bottle. Close the bottle tightly and keep it closed until you are ready to use the blend.

2. Before bed, place 5 drops of the oil blend on a cotton swab or cotton ball and rub over your acne. Leave it on for 5 minutes, then dab off any excess with a tissue.

3. Apply nightly until the acne fades. Store the remaining blend in a cool place out of direct sunlight.

Aging Skin

Excessive sun exposure, smoking, or a diet low in antioxidants can all cause skin to age sooner and more rapidly than we would like. The astringent and regenerative properties of essential oils can renew your skin and help slow the aging process. I've chosen sweet almond oil and jojoba oil for carrier oils because of their soft texture, moisturizing effects, and pleasant scents.

AGING SKIN TIGHTENING RUB

Makes 4 to 8 treatments

2 tablespoons sweet almond oil
12 drops sandalwood essential oil
8 drops geranium essential oil

1. In a small glass or metal bowl, combine the sweet almond oil with the sandalwood and geranium essential oils. Store in a 1-ounce dark amber or cobalt glass bottle.

2. After cleansing your skin, smooth 1 teaspoon of this blend onto your face and neck.

3. Use once daily. Store the remaining blend in a cool place out of direct sunlight.

Makes 6 to 9 treatments

6 tablespoons jojoba oil
30 drops myrrh essential oil

1. In a 4-ounce dark amber or cobalt glass jar, combine the jojoba oil and myrrh essential oil. Cap the jar and shake well to combine.

2. Using the tip of your finger, or with a cotton swab, gently apply a few drops to the skin under your eyes and massage until the oil is absorbed.

3. Use once daily. Store the remaining blend in a cool place out of direct sunlight.

Air Freshener

How does that stale smell come into your home? If you have to keep windows closed during a long winter, you can still freshen the air indoors with essential oils. A simple mix of these oils with water will provide enough natural deodorizing power to keep you from spending money on perfumed chemical-based air fresheners.

PINE AIR FRESHENER SPRAY

Makes 16 ounces

2 cups water
16 drops eucalyptus essential oil
16 drops pine essential oil
16 drops tea tree essential oil

1. In a pint-size glass or metal spray bottle, combine the water with the eucalyptus, pine, and tea tree essential oils. Cap the bottle and shake well to combine.

2. Mist this freshener around your house wherever—and whenever—it will do some good.

3. Store the remaining blend in a cool place out of direct sunlight.

NOTE: In addition to the essential oils used in this recipe, many other essential oil combinations will work, too: lemon and eucalyptus for a clean scent, or orange, clove, and sandalwood for warm, bright notes.

Anger

How often do we hear that we should step back and take a deep breath when something makes us angry? Here's a way to make that pause to breathe as effective as possible: Scent it with the calming effects of aromatherapy. These recipes will help you find the fragrances that bring you back to earth, whether you use them at home, in the car, or at the office.

ANGER DIFFUSER TREATMENT

Makes 1 diffusion

3 drops chamomile (German or Roman) essential oil
3 drops balsam fir essential oil
3 drops rose essential oil
3 drops sandalwood essential oil

To the water in your diffuser, add the chamomile, balsam fir, rose, and sandalwood essential oils, and turn it on. Let the diffuser run for at least 15 minutes. Breathe.

ANGER SPRAY BLEND

Makes 1 ounce

2 tablespoons distilled water
3 drops lavender essential oil
1 drop clary sage essential oil
1 drop galbanum essential oil
1 drop peppermint essential oil

1. In a 1-ounce glass or metal spray bottle, combine the water with the lavender, clary sage, galbanum, and peppermint essential oils. Cap the bottle and shake well to combine.

continued >

2. Spray this blend at home, in the car, or use it (judiciously) in an area of your workplace where you can enjoy it without objection from your coworkers. If you have an office with a door, close the door before spraying.

3. Store the remaining blend in a cool place out of direct sunlight until you need it again.

Anxiety

Many essential oils can help ease the anxiousness that comes with daily work and life. The solutions suggested here can bring relaxation and release when the day's events overwhelm your sense of well-being. Milk aids the oils' absorption into the bath water, so they don't float on top.

ANXIETY-RELEASING BATH

Makes 1 treatment

½ cup milk
4 drops sandalwood essential oil
1 drop ylang-ylang essential oil

1. In a small glass or metal bowl, mix the milk with the sandalwood and ylang-ylang essential oils.

2. Run a warm bath and then add the milk and oils to the warm water.

3. Step in, breathe in the scents, and relax.

ANXIETY-REDUCING SPRAY

Makes 2 ounces

4 tablespoons distilled water
6 drops lavender essential oil
2 drops cedarwood essential oil
2 drops geranium essential oil
2 drops spearmint essential oil

1. In a 4-ounce glass or metal spray bottle, mix the water with the lavender, cedarwood, geranium, and spearmint essential oils. Cap the bottle and shake well to combine.

2. Spray 2 or 3 pumps in your home or car, as needed.

3. Store the remaining blend in a cool place out of direct sunlight. Remember to shake again before each use.

Arthritis

Wherever the pain of arthritis strikes, a topical application of essential oils with their anti-inflammatory properties can help bring relief to stiff, aching joints. Clove and sandalwood essential oils can also provide penetrating pain relief. In addition to Biblical essential oils, add evening primrose, a carrier oil that is one of nature's most effective anti-inflammatory oils. If evening primrose is not available, jojoba oil or sweet almond oil are good substitutes.

ARTHRITIS PAIN RELIEF RUB

Makes 6 treatments

2 tablespoons evening primrose oil
15 drops clove essential oil
15 drops sandalwood essential oil

1. In a 2-ounce dark amber or cobalt glass bottle, mix the evening primrose oil with the clove and sandalwood essential oils. Cap the bottle and shake well to combine.

2. Apply about 1 teaspoon of this mixture directly to the affected area and massage it into the skin.

3. Repeat as needed for pain. Store the remaining blend in a cool place out of direct sunlight.

Makes 12 treatments

4 tablespoons evening primrose oil
24 drops eucalyptus essential oil
24 drops balsam fir essential oil
12 drops spearmint essential oil

1. In a 4-ounce dark amber or cobalt glass bottle, mix the evening primrose oil with the eucalyptus, balsam fir, and spearmint essential oils. Cap the bottle and shake well to combine.

2. Apply 1 teaspoon of this mixture directly to the affected area and massage it into the skin.

3. Store the remaining blend in a cool place out of direct sunlight.

Asthma

Nothing is more frightening than watching your child with asthma struggle to breathe, or to feel the restriction in your own airway. Essential oils can help relieve asthma symptoms through inhalation, especially when activated with heat. An asthma attack can be life threatening, so if using these methods does not improve breathing, use your prescription medications and seek the help of your physician or visit an emergency room, as needed. You can still use the following methods to supplement your doctor's instructions, but restoring breathing is the first priority.

ASTHMA STEAM RELIEF

Makes 1 treatment

3 cups water
¼ teaspoon (25 drops) eucalyptus essential oil

1. In a small pot over high heat, heat the water until it simmers.

2. Turn off the heat and add the eucalyptus essential oil.

3. Place a trivet or hot pad on a surface you can bend your head over. Place the pot on the trivet. Cover your head with a towel and bend over the steaming water, using the towel to trap the steam. Breathe deeply.

4. Come up for fresh air when you need it, and continue to breathe the steam until the water cools.

5. Do this as often as you like, refreshing the water with new hot water and eucalyptus essential oil.

NOTE: You can substitute lavender or peppermint essential oil for the eucalyptus.

ASTHMA VAPOR RUB

Makes 4 treatments

¼ cup olive oil
12 drops lavender essential oil
8 drops geranium essential oil
2 drops frankincense essential oil
2 drops peppermint essential oil

1. In a 4-ounce dark amber or cobalt glass bottle, combine the olive oil with the lavender, geranium, frankincense, and peppermint essential oils. Cap the bottle and shake well to combine.

2. Rub about 1 tablespoon of the mixture onto the chest. This remedy is particularly effective just before bedtime, so after application, cover up with an old t-shirt or a pajama shirt.

3. Store the remaining blend in a cool place out of direct sunlight.

Back Pain

If you know your back pain comes from the hours you spend standing at work, the new workout you took on a little too enthusiastically, or the way-too-late night you spent at the keyboard, these remedies will help loosen your muscles and take the edge off the pain. If, however, you have a ruptured disk or serious injury, see your doctor before you begin any alternative care plan.

BACK PAIN RUB

Makes 3 to 4 treatments

2 tablespoons olive oil
10 drops balsam poplar essential oil
10 drops rosemary essential oil
6 drops lavender essential oil
4 drops cassia essential oil
4 drops eucalyptus essential oil

1. In a small glass or metal bowl, mix the olive oil with the balsam poplar, rosemary, lavender, cassia, and eucalyptus essential oils.
2. Rub (or have someone rub) some of the blend into your sore back muscles.
3. Do this twice daily until the pain subsides. Store the remaining blend in a 1-ounce dark amber or cobalt glass bottle in a cool place out of direct sunlight.

BACK PAIN SOAK

Makes 1 treatment

½ cup Epsom salt
10 drops clary sage essential oil
10 drops lavender essential oil

1. In a small glass or metal bowl, use a spoon to combine the Epsom salt with the clary sage and lavender essential oils.

2. Run a warm bath. Add the salt mixture to the water all at once and swish the water around to dissolve the salt.

3. Soak in the tub for 15 to 20 minutes.

Bathroom Care

If the smells of ammonia and chlorine do not appeal to you, several essential oils and odorless baking soda can change the way you clean and disinfect your bathroom.

BATHROOM GROUT SPRAY

Makes 16 ounces

2 cups water
2 teaspoons (200 drops) tea tree essential oil

1. In a pint-size glass or metal spray bottle, mix the water and tea tree essential oil. Cap the bottle and shake well to combine.

2. Spritz the mixture on grout or caulking that has mildewed. Don't rinse it—let it work away at the stains. Repeat as needed to defeat mildew and mold.

3. Store the remaining blend in a cool place out of direct sunlight.

BATHTUB CLEANER

Makes 1 application

1 cup baking soda
24 drops grapefruit essential oil
24 drops tea tree essential oil

1. In a medium glass or metal bowl, mix the baking soda with the grapefruit and tea tree essential oils.

2. Sprinkle this powder on your tub and scrub it with a sponge or brush.

3. Rinse with water. The waxy soap buildup will rinse away.

Makes 20 ounces (6 to 10 uses)

2¼ cups water
¼ cup unscented liquid castile soap
4 drops lavender essential oil
4 drops lemon essential oil
4 drops tea tree essential oil

1. In a 32-ounce glass or metal spray bottle, combine the water, castile soap, and the lavender, lemon, and tea tree essential oils. Cap the bottle and shake well to combine.
2. Spray this in your toilet bowl and scrub it with a brush.
3. Flush to rinse. Store the remaining blend in a cool place out of direct sunlight.

Blisters

When fluid is trapped under your skin, it forms a blister, like a bubble on the surface. Blisters can be painful when they burst, and the underlying tissue can become infected. Sometimes these bubbles form as a result of herpes simplex or athlete's foot. Here's how to keep them from becoming more than a nuisance.

BLISTER DISINFECTING TREATMENT

Makes 5 treatments

10 drops carrier oil of choice
5 drops benzoin (onycha) essential oil
5 drops lavender essential oil
5 drops myrtle essential oil

1. In a small (5-mL) dark amber or cobalt glass bottle, add the carrier oil followed by the benzoin, lavender, and myrtle essential oils. Cap the bottle and shake well to combine.

2. Apply about 5 drops to a cotton swab and gently pat the broken skin, getting the oil under the broken skin and in contact with the exposed layer.

3. Cover with an adhesive bandage or use a doughnut-shaped moleskin to protect the area if you need to wear shoes.

4. Apply twice daily until the blistered skin closes. Store the remaining blend in a cool place out of direct sunlight.

BLISTER INTERIM CARE

Makes 1 treatment

1 to 2 drops German chamomile or frankincense essential oil

1. Once the dead skin has lifted naturally away from the blistered spot, carefully trim it off.

2. Treat the new skin underneath with 1 to 2 drops of essential oil daily until it toughens.

Bloating

The mild to severe discomfort of bloating can be a symptom of many things: general indigestion, food allergies or sensitivities, bowel obstruction, or even serious disease. Lemon essential oil acts as a natural diuretic, which can help get things moving again; coriander and peppermint have properties that relieve gas and bloating. If time and the natural remedy provided here do not relieve the situation, seek the help of your physician.

BLOATING RELIEF RUB

Makes 1 treatment

6 drops olive oil
2 drops coriander essential oil
2 drops lemon essential oil
2 drops peppermint essential oil

continued >

1. In a small glass or metal bowl, stir together the olive oil with the coriander, lemon, and peppermint essential oils.

2. With your fingertips, apply the blend in a clockwise direction to the abdomen.

3. Lie on your left side for 15 minutes. Breathe in the scents of the essential oils to expand their effectiveness and help you relax.

Body Odor

Body odor comes from bacteria that thrive on the body when you perspire, so people who are more physically active are more likely to produce an odor. You can use body sprays and commercial deodorants to combat this, but essential oils provide a natural option that may be a better fit for your lifestyle.

DEODORANT SPRAY

Makes 3 ounces (5 to 6 applications)

6 tablespoons grain alcohol
30 drops tea tree essential oil

1. In a 4-ounce glass or metal spray bottle, mix the alcohol with the tea tree essential oil. Cap the bottle and shake well to combine.

2. Spray this on your clean armpits after you shower. Store the remaining blend in a cool place out of direct sunlight.

NOTE: For the grain alcohol, I recommend Everclear. In addition to the tea tree essential oil used in this recipe, lavender, lemon, pine, or spearmint essential oils are also antibacterial, and will work well if you prefer one of these scents.

DEODORANT STICK

Makes 1 deodorant stick

¼ cup aluminum-free baking soda
¼ cup arrowroot or cornstarch
5 drops of one of the following antibacterial essential oils:
 cumin essential oil
 geranium essential oil
 lavender essential oil
 lemon essential oil
 lime essential oil
 pine essential oil
 spearmint essential oil
 thyme essential oil
3 to 5 tablespoons coconut oil
1 empty stick deodorant container

1. In a small glass or metal bowl, mix the baking soda and arrowroot with the essential oil of choice.

2. One tablespoon at a time, add the coconut oil and blend with a pastry blender until fully blended into a paste consistency. Press this into your deodorant container and let stand until the coconut oil solidifies.

3. Apply as needed. Store the remaining blend in a cool place out of direct sunlight.

DEODORANT STICK FOR HOT CLIMATES

Makes 1 deodorant stick

1½ teaspoons grapeseed oil
¾ teaspoon shea butter
¾ teaspoon vegetable glycerin
1 tablespoon baking soda
3 drops cassie essential oil or absolute
3 drops eucalyptus essential oil
3 drops peppermint essential oil
3 drops pine essential oil
3 drops cistus essential oil

continued >

1. In a small glass or metal bowl, combine the grapeseed oil, shea butter, and glycerin.
2. Microwave for 10 seconds on high, or until the shea butter melts.
3. Stir in the baking soda and the cassie, eucalyptus, peppermint, pine, and cistus essential oils. Pour the mixture into an empty deodorant container.
4. Refrigerate until it solidifies, and keep refrigerated between uses.

NOTE: This deodorant is especially good for use in warm climates because the shea butter works to combat odor in high heat.

Bronchitis

When the respiratory system becomes inflamed with the respiratory disease known as bronchitis, it produces excess mucus and long spasms of coughing. Bronchitis can worsen and lead to pneumonia, and it can be an indicator of a more serious condition such as chronic obstructive pulmonary disease. Eucalyptus and rosemary are both effective at opening constricted bronchial passages, so direct treatment can be helpful. If your case does not respond to these treatments in one to two days, seek the advice of your physician.

BRONCHITIS EUCALYPTUS DIFFUSION

Makes 1 diffusion

5 drops eucalyptus essential oil

1. To a diffuser, add the eucalyptus essential oil. Take the diffuser into a contained space such as a closed bedroom.
2. Turn on the diffuser and let it run until all the oil has diffused.

BRONCHITIS STEAM TREATMENT

Makes 1 treatment

3 cups water

¼ teaspoon (25 drops) eucalyptus or rosemary essential oil

1. In a small saucepan over high heat, heat the water to a simmer.

2. Turn off the heat and add the eucalyptus essential oil.

3. Place a trivet or a hot pad on a surface you can bend your head over. Place the pot on the trivet. Cover your head with a towel and bend over the steaming water, using the towel to trap the steam. Breathe deeply.

4. Come up for fresh air when you need it, and continue to breathe the steam until the water cools.

5. Do this as often as you like, refreshing the water with new hot water and essential oil.

Bug Bites and Stings

When mosquitoes bite and the bites become itchy, we want relief as quickly as we can get it. Essential oils with anti-itch properties can solve this problem in minutes, and they can be applied as often as necessary until the bumps disappear. Bee stings are a more serious issue—they can cause pain, fever, and even headaches, and people who are allergic to them can have more dangerous reactions. If the stinger remains in the wound, it can create greater pain and swelling. Check first with a magnifying glass and remove the stinger with tweezers, or by scraping with a credit card. When the stinger is gone, apply an essential oil that has antihistamine and anti-inflammatory properties.

NEAT BUG BITE ITCH TREATMENT

Makes 1 treatment

1 drop lavender, peppermint, or wintergreen essential oil

1. Apply 1 drop of the essential oil of choice directly on the sting every 15 minutes for the first hour after the sting. All 3 oils listed have antipruritic (anti-itch) properties, so they will ease the discomfort of the insect sting.

2. After the first hour, apply 1 drop of any one of these oils 3 times daily until the sting stops bothering you.

BEE STING COLD COMPRESS

Makes 1 treatment

2 cups cold water
10 drops galbanum essential oil
1 drop chamomile (German or Roman) essential oil

1. In a medium glass or metal bowl or a low basin, mix the water and galbanum essential oil.

2. Soak a hand towel in the water, allowing it to absorb the liquid.

3. Wring out the towel and place it on the bee sting. Wrap it in place using a second hand towel and plastic wrap.

4. If you can, leave this on for several hours (change the compress with a fresh one as it gets warm), and you will defeat the swelling and quell the pain.

5. Once you remove the compress, apply 1 drop of undiluted chamomile essential oil, 3 times a day, directly on the sting location.

Bug Repellent

Here you'll find information for keeping mosquitoes and other biting insects at bay. Citronella is well known as an effective mosquito repellent, and you can buy candles, lamp oil, and a number of other products that dispense it. In the first remedy below, it gets a boost from a number of nature's other effective oils. While few substances are as effective at chasing away mosquitoes as the chemical known as DEET, citronella is also scientifically proven to ward off insects, especially when mixed with pure vanilla extract (the same kind you use in baking—but make sure it's pure vanilla and not imitation). It has a shorter interval of effectiveness than DEET, however, so reapply at least every three hours.

NATURAL INSECT REPELLENT

Makes 2 or 3 applications

2 tablespoons grain alcohol or rubbing alcohol
12 drops citronella essential oil
12 drops eucalyptus essential oil
6 drops cedarwood essential oil
6 drops geranium essential oil

1. In a small glass or metal bowl, mix the alcohol with the citronella, eucalyptus, cedarwood, and geranium essential oils. Stir to combine well. Transfer to a 2-ounce glass or metal spray bottle.

2. Apply sparingly to your skin, as this is highly concentrated.

3. Use as needed on clothing (except silk, which will be stained on contact) and on the brim of your hat rather than applying all over your skin.

4. Store any remaining repellent in a 1-ounce dark amber or cobalt glass bottle in a cool place out of direct sunlight until you need it again.

NOTE: For the grain alcohol, I recommend Everclear.

Makes 8 ounces

1 cup water
1 tablespoon pure vanilla extract
6 drops lavender essential oil
4 drops lemongrass essential oil
3 drops citronella essential oil
2 drops ginger essential oil

1. In a 12-ounce glass or metal spray bottle, combine the water with the vanilla extract and the lavender, lemongrass, citronella, and ginger essential oils. Cap the bottle and shake well to combine.

2. Spray on your skin and clothing (but not silk, which will be stained on contact), and around the brim of your hat. **Do not spray on your face**.

3. Repeat as needed to deter mosquitoes. Store the remaining blend in a cool place out of direct sunlight.

Cellulite

Women tend to have more body fat than men do, and a woman's skin has a thinner outer layer than a man's skin. When the fat packets in women's skin just below the epidermis become enlarged, they become the visible "cottage cheese" skin we know as cellulite. Sadly, no method has been discovered that makes cellulite disappear, but some essential oils can help break it down and make it less visible.

DAILY CELLULITE MASSAGE

Makes 8 ounces (10 to 14 treatments)

1 cup grapeseed oil
20 drops fennel essential oil
20 drops juniper essential oil

10 drops of one of the following:
    cypress essential oil
    grapefruit essential oil
    lemon essential oil
    rosemary essential oil
    sage essential oil

1. In a small glass or metal bowl, combine the grapeseed oil with the fennel and juniper essential oils, and the essential oil of choice. Mix well.

2. Before you use the massage oil, use a dry body brush (such as a sisal brush) to gently brush the cellulite-stricken areas of your body until your skin is pink.

3. Daily, massage the oil into your cellulite areas for 10 minutes to diminish its appearance.

4. Store the remaining mixture in a dark amber or cobalt glass bottle or jar in a cool place out of direct sunlight.

CELLULITE HELICHRYSUM TREATMENT

Makes 1 treatment

1 tablespoon olive oil
5 drops helichrysum essential oil

1. In a small glass or metal bowl, mix the olive oil and helichrysum essential oil.

2. Daily, massage this blend into your problem cellulite areas until it is absorbed into your skin and you see results.

NOTE: Helichrysum essential oil is a natural anti-inflammatory, making it effective for a wide range of skin issues. If you're not seeing the results you want from your daily massage (and you've already taken off some weight and you're getting regular exercise), try adding this to your daily regimen.

Chapped Lips

Whether you live in a climate with six months of bitter winter or in the bone-dry desert, you know what discomfort chapped lips can create. These simple remedies give you moisturizing relief along with the regenerative powers of essential oils. Which one you use is entirely a matter of personal preference; some people prefer the clear, shiny aloe vera gel on their lips, while others like the richness of shea butter.

CHAPPED LIPS GEL

Makes 1 treatment

1 large drop aloe vera gel
1 drop frankincense or myrrh essential oil

1. Place 1 drop of aloe vera gel on your index finger.
2. Add 1 drop of your essential oil of choice.
3. Smooth between your finger and thumb to mix.
4. Apply to your lips. Repeat as often as you like to fight dryness and chapping.

SHEA BUTTER FOR CHAPPED LIPS

Makes 1 treatment

1 fingertip's worth of shea butter (about ¼ teaspoon)
1 drop cistus essential oil

1. Place the shea butter on your index finger.
2. Add 1 drop of cistus essential oil.
3. Smooth between your finger and thumb to mix.
4. Apply to your lips. Repeat as often as you like to fight dryness and chapping.

NOTE: If you don't have cistus essential oil, lavender, myrrh, or frankincense essential oil will work.

Chilblains

If you've been exposed to cold, damp conditions for long periods, you may know the discomfort of chilblains—also known as pernio. The small, swollen, itchy spots on fingers, toes, ears, and nose are not life threatening, but they can be a nuisance.

CHILBLAINS LAYERING TREATMENT

Makes 1 treatment

1 drop myrrh essential oil
1 drop lavender essential oil
1 drop helichrysum essential oil
3 drops sweet almond oil

1. Using your fingertips, apply the myrrh essential oil to the affected area.
2. Next, apply the lavender essential oil on top of the myrrh.
3. Now apply the helichrysum essential oil over the lavender.
4. Top these with the sweet almond oil.
5. Repeat this up to 4 times daily until the chilblains are healed.

SOOTHING SANDALWOOD AND CEDARWOOD BATH FOR CHILBLAINS

Makes 5 treatments

5 tablespoons calendula oil
6 drops cedarwood essential oil
6 drops lavender essential oil
6 drops sandalwood essential oil

1. In a 4-ounce dark amber or cobalt glass bottle, combine the calendula oil with the cedarwood, lavender, and sandalwood essential oils. Cap the bottle and shake well to combine.
2. Run a warm bath and, while the water is running, add 1 tablespoon of the blend to the warm water.

continued >

3. Soak for at least 15 minutes.

4. Repeat daily until the chilblains are healed.

5. Store the remaining bath oil in a cool place out of direct sunlight.

Colds and Flu

Sneezing, sniffles, upper respiratory congestion, coughing, and low-grade fever are all common symptoms of the world's most ubiquitous and contagious malady. There's no cure for the common cold and no easy way to fight the flu, but you can arm yourself against the next onslaught by keeping some antiviral and symptom-fighting essential oils on hand, including eucalyptus, fir, frankincense, lavender, lemon, myrrh, myrtle, spearmint, and tea tree.

COLD- AND FLU-FIGHTING STEAM

Makes 1 treatment

1 to 1½ cups steaming-hot water
1 drop balsam fir essential oil
1 drop lavender essential oil
1 drop myrrh essential oil
1 drop tea tree essential oil

1. Into a medium glass or metal bowl set on a heatproof surface, pour the hot water.

2. Add the balsam fir, lavender, myrrh, and tea tree essential oils.

3. Place a trivet or hot pad on a surface you can bend your head over. Place the bowl on the trivet. Cover your head with a towel and bend over the steaming water, using the towel to trap the steam. Breathe deeply.

4. Come up for fresh air when you need it, and continue to breathe the steam until the water cools.

5. Repeat this process as often as you wish.

VAPOR RUB FOR COLDS AND FLU

Makes 5 treatments

2 tablespoons sweet almond oil or jojoba oil
15 drops rosemary essential oil
10 drops eucalyptus essential oil
5 drops lemon essential oil

1. In a 2-ounce dark amber or cobalt glass bottle, combine the sweet almond oil with the rosemary, eucalyptus, and lemon essential oils.
2. Gently rub this blend on your chest, neck, cheekbones, and around your nose, following the line of your sinus cavities.
3. Repeat 2 to 3 times daily until your symptoms clear. Store the remaining blend in a cool place out of direct sunlight.

Colic

When your baby cries uncontrollably for hours at a time, and continues to cry like this more than three days a week for several weeks in a row, she has colic—and you have sleepless nights and high stress levels. The condition is not permanent, but no parent can bear to hear their baby cry without doing something to soothe her.

COLIC MASSAGE

Makes 1 treatment

1 teaspoon sweet almond oil
1 drop geranium essential oil
1 drop lavender essential oil

1. In your palm, mix the sweet almond oil with the geranium and lavender essential oils until they are warm.
2. Using a little of the oil on your fingertips, gently rub this blend in a circular, clockwise motion on your baby's stomach.
3. When the baby becomes quieter, turn him over onto his stomach and continue the gentle massage on his back.

Makes 1 compress

2 cups warm water
1 drop lavender essential oil

1. In a small glass or metal bowl, combine the water and lavender essential oil.
2. Place a washcloth on the surface of the water and let it become saturated.
3. Lift the washcloth from the water and wring out the excess water.
4. As your baby lies on her back, place the wet compress on her stomach. Once the compress cools to the point it no longer keeps your baby warm and comfortable, remove it.
5. If the crying begins again, repeat the process.

Conjunctivitis

Conjunctivitis, or "pink eye," is an infection of the transparent membrane covering the white part of the eye. Not only is it irritating, it's also highly contagious, and children often pass it from one to the next. You can take steps to relieve the itching and soreness using warm compresses and rose essential oil, but anything you use must be disinfected immediately to keep from spreading the infection to others in the family.

CONJUNCTIVITIS COMPRESS

Makes 1 compress

2 cups warm water
5 drops rose essential oil

1. In a small glass or metal bowl, combine the water and rose essential oil.
2. Place a washcloth on the surface of the water and let it become saturated.

3. Lift the washcloth from the water and wring out the excess water.

4. Place the wet compress over the affected eye. (It may be easiest to have your child lie down for this, or for you to lie down if you're the one affected.)

5. When the compress cools to the point it no longer feels warm, remove it. Immediately wash out the compress with soap and hot water, and wash your hands, as well.

6. Repeat as often as you wish. If the condition doesn't clear up in 2 to 3 days, see your doctor. The infection may be bacterial rather than viral, and antibiotics may be required.

Cough

Colds, allergies, and post-nasal drip can create a nagging tickle that just doesn't seem to go away. Cough drops made with honey or horehound can be effective natural remedies. While *no essential oil should be taken internally,* you can soothe the cough using your vaporizer and a range of essential oils—and throat and chest rubs can penetrate to help clear the source of the tickle.

CHEST RUB FOR COUGH

Makes 5 treatments

2 tablespoons olive oil
15 drops eucalyptus essential oil
10 drops balsam fir essential oil

1. In a 2-ounce dark amber or cobalt glass bottle or jar, combine the olive oil with the eucalyptus and balsam fir essential oils.

2. Rub this blend over your chest and throat.

3. Repeat as desired. Store the remaining blend in a cool place out of direct sunlight.

COUGH CONGESTION-BUSTING VAPOR

Makes 1 treatment

3 drops each of 1 or more of the following:
    chamomile essential oil (German or Roman)
    frankincense essential oil
    ginger essential oil
    lavender essential oil
    oregano essential oil
    sandalwood essential oil
    tea tree essential oil

1. To the water in your vaporizer, add the essential oils of choice, and turn it on.

2. Stay in the room with the vaporizer running for at least 15 minutes every hour.

3. Repeat as often as you wish.

Cradle Cap

It looks potentially worrisome to new parents, but cradle cap is a very common ailment that children grow out of after the age of one. The crust of dead skin cells can be remedied with a simple balm that kills bacteria when gently massaged into your baby's scalp.

CRADLE CAP SCALP TREATMENT

Makes 1 treatment

1 teaspoon jojoba oil
2 drops geranium or rose geranium essential oil

1. In your palm, combine the jojoba oil with the geranium essential oil. Rub both palms together to warm the oils.

2. Gently apply the blend to your baby's scalp. Be careful not to get any of the oil in his eyes.

3. With a baby brush, gently rub the oil into the affected area.

4. Repeat this 3 times daily until the condition clears.

Cuts and Scrapes

Use the antiseptic and antibacterial qualities of essential oils in place of commercial first-aid creams for minor cuts and scrapes. Many essential oils can prevent infection and allow your wound to heal naturally and effectively, without the sting of an alcohol-based disinfectant.

WASH FOR MINOR CUTS

Makes 1 treatment

Warm water
3 drops of one of the following:
    eucalyptus essential oil
    lavender essential oil
    lemon essential oil
    pine essential oil
    sandalwood essential oil
    spikenard essential oil
    tea tree essential oil

1. Fill a sink or large glass or metal bowl with warm water.

2. Add 3 drops of the essential oil of choice.

3. Bathe the cut or scrape in the water, then dry with a clean towel.

NEAT TREATMENT FOR CUTS AND SCRAPES

Makes 1 treatment

1 or 2 drops of one of the following antibacterial essential oils:
    eucalyptus essential oil
    lavender essential oil
    lemon essential oil
    pine essential oil
    sandalwood essential oil
    spikenard essential oil
    tea tree essential oil

continued >

1. Place 1 or 2 drops of the essential oil of choice directly on the cut or scrape.

2. If there is a chance the wound could pick up dirt or could be reinjured, use sterile materials to bandage the cut or scrape.

3. Change the bandage daily, and reapply the essential oil, neat, with each new bandage.

NOTE: Eucalyptus, lavender, and tea tree essential oils are all soothing, as well as good shields against infection.

Diaper Rash

If you don't like the idea of using commercial diaper rash products on your baby's sensitive skin, essential oils provide an alternative. Here are options that will cool the rash and bring comfort to your baby.

SOOTHING DIAPER RASH WASH

Makes 20 treatments

10 drops lavender essential oil
10 drops yarrow essential oil
2 cups warm water

1. In a small (5-mL) dark amber or cobalt glass bottle, blend the lavender and yarrow essential oils. Cap the bottle and shake well to combine.

2. In a medium glass or metal bowl, combine the water with 1 drop of the lavender-yarrow essential oil blend.

3. Soak a soft cloth in the warm water, wring it out, and use it to cleanse your baby.

4. Dry the diaper area and use a cotton ball to apply additional oil-treated water to your baby's bottom.

5. Store the remaining oil blend in a cool place out of direct sunlight until needed.

DIAPER RASH PROTECTION

Makes 20 treatments

10 drops lavender essential oil
10 drops yarrow essential oil
4 teaspoons sweet almond oil or jojoba oil

1. In a small (5-mL) dark amber or cobalt glass bottle, blend the lavender and yarrow essential oils. Cap the bottle and shake well to combine.

2. In your palm, mix the sweet almond oil with 1 drop of the lavender-yarrow essential oil blend.

3. Smooth a light layer of this protective oil over the diaper area before putting on a new diaper.

4. Store the remaining blend in a cool place out of direct sunlight until needed.

Diarrhea

The clinical definition of diarrhea includes watery bowel movements of abnormal frequency—say, every hour or so for several hours or longer. An intestinal disorder of this kind can make you pass a quart of liquid in a day, so drinking lots of water (or sports drinks that supply the electrolyte balance you need) is the most important thing you can do. Diarrhea that lasts two days or more becomes a health risk because of the danger of dehydration. If you frequently experience loose stools that you can't connect to a stomach virus or food poisoning, you may have a chronic condition that requires medical intervention. If your diarrhea does not begin to clear up after four days, consult your doctor.

Makes 3 treatments

1 tablespoon olive oil
9 drops lavender essential oil
3 drops cedarwood essential oil
3 drops eucalyptus essential oil
3 drops tea tree essential oil

1. In a 1-ounce dark amber or cobalt glass bottle, combine the olive oil with the lavender, cedarwood, eucalyptus, and tea tree essential oils. Cap the bottle and shake well to combine.

2. Apply 1 teaspoon to your abdomen, massaging it in a circular, clockwise motion until the oils are absorbed.

3. Repeat as needed after each episode of diarrhea. Store the remaining blend in a cool place out of direct sunlight.

Ear Infection

Not every earache is an infection. Some come from a buildup of fluid in the ear, which becomes painful when the pressure increases during a cold or when seasonal allergies flare up. When pain persists even when the sinus congestion has cleared, there may be an infection present, and if the pain continues for more than a few hours, it's time to have a doctor take a look inside. Ear infections can cause long-term complications, especially in children. If you have a baby or toddler who keeps holding or pulling on one ear and you can see redness inside, call your doctor.

EAR INFECTION OLIVE OIL REMEDY

Makes 4 treatments

1 tablespoon warm olive oil
2 drops cedarwood essential oil
2 drops lavender essential oil
2 drops Roman chamomile essential oil
2 drops rosemary essential oil

1. In a 1-ounce dark amber or cobalt glass bottle, mix the olive oil with the cedarwood, lavender, Roman chamomile, and rosemary essential oils. Cap the bottle and shake well to combine.

2. With a cotton swab, apply the oil around the opening of the ear, around the outside of the ear, and on the earlobe.

3. Place a warm compress (such as a folded washcloth soaked in warm water and wrung nearly dry) over the affected ear to warm the oils and help them penetrate.

4. Repeat every 2 hours until the pressure subsides. If the pain continues for more than 6 hours, consult a doctor.

5. Store the remaining blend in a cool place out of direct sunlight.

EAR INFECTION COTTON REMEDY

Makes 1 treatment

3 drops lavender essential oil

1. Place the lavender essential oil on a cotton ball, and place this over the ear opening.

2. Leave it in place overnight.

Eczema

Eczema presents as red, itchy, peeling patches of skin that arise in a multitude of situations, from using a new soap or detergent to enduring a period of prolonged stress. When you find yourself scratching where you usually don't scratch, reach for your essential oils to calm the inflammation.

ECZEMA ANTI-ITCH BLEND

Makes 3 to 5 treatments

1 tablespoon coconut oil
2 drops frankincense essential oil
2 drops helichrysum essential oil
1 drop geranium essential oil
1 drop thyme essential oil

continued >

1. In a small glass or metal bowl, mix the coconut oil with the frankincense, helichrysum, geranium, and thyme essential oils.

2. With your fingers, apply this blend to the itchy areas.

3. Cover the treated area with gauze. If the area is on your hand or foot, put on white cotton gloves or cotton socks. Keep the area covered throughout the day. If you must remove the gauze or gloves, reapply the treatment, up to 3 times per day.

4. Repeat as needed until the itching stops.

5. Store any unused blend in a small (5-mL) dark amber or cobalt glass bottle in a cool place out of direct sunlight.

Fatigue

If you prefer to battle that 3 p.m. drowsiness with a natural remedy instead of an energy drink, your essential oils can help. The best cure for fatigue is sleep, of course, but that's not practical in the middle of the workday or if your evening is loaded with your children's activities. Here are some remedies to help you keep moving when your eyelids have other ideas.

FATIGUE-FIGHTING DIFFUSION

Makes 4 diffusions

4 drops anise essential oil
4 drops cassia essential oil
3 drops cinnamon essential oil
3 drops pine essential oil
2 drops bdellium essential oil

1. In a small (5-mL) dark amber or cobalt glass bottle, mix the anise, cassia, cinnamon, pine, and bdellium essential oils. Cap the bottle and shake well to combine.

2. Add 4 drops of this blend to your diffuser, and run the diffuser for 15 minutes in your car or office (if you have one with a door), or at home.

3. Cap the jar tightly and store any remaining oil blend in a cool place out of direct sunlight.

STIMULATING AIR FRESHENER

Makes 10 applications

3 tablespoons distilled water or spring water
3 tablespoons vodka or grain alcohol
12 drops peppermint essential oil
12 drops lemon essential oil
6 drops frankincense essential oil

1. In a 4-ounce glass or metal spray bottle, mix the water and vodka with the peppermint, lemon, and frankincense essential oils. Cap the bottle and shake well to combine.

2. Spray this in your room or car once every 2 hours, as needed. Store the remaining blend in a cool place out of direct sunlight.

NOTE: Any brand of vodka will do but for the grain alcohol, I recommend Everclear.

Fever

The symptoms caused by fever can make you miserable: dizziness, lack of appetite, alternating chills and sweating, fatigue, and muscle aches. A number of essential oils (any of the mint oils, as well as bay and cassia) can help reduce a fever through their overall cooling effects. If the ill person is a child, review the precautions of the following recipe before treating young children.

FEVER-COOLING NEAT TREATMENT

Makes 1 treatment

3 or 4 drops peppermint essential oil

1. Place the peppermint essential oil on a cotton ball.
2. Apply the oil directly to the back of the neck and the soles of the feet.
3. Repeat this every 30 minutes until the fever goes down.

CAUTIONARY NOTE: Peppermint essential oil should not be used with children under 7 years of age. If your child is 7 or older, it will need to be diluted. Dilute 1 or 2 drops of peppermint essential oil in 1 tablespoon of a carrier oil of your choice before applying it to your child's skin.

FEVER-REDUCING COLD PACK

Makes 1 treatment

1 cup cold water
3 drops spearmint essential oil
1 drop eucalyptus essential oil

1. In a small glass or metal bowl, mix the water with the spearmint and eucalyptus essential oils.
2. Place a hand towel or a cloth bandage on the surface of the water and let it become saturated.
3. Remove the towel and wring out any excess water.
4. Place the cold compress on the forehead. Cover it with a plastic bag or sheet of plastic wrap to contain the moisture. Hold the compress and plastic in place with a hand towel, or tie it in place with an elastic bandage, just tight enough to hold the compress.
5. When the compress warms to body temperature, replace it with another cold compress. Repeat until the fever is reduced.

Flatulence

If you feel bloated, crampy, and generally uncomfortable and you feel like you're expelling a lot of gas, you are not alone. Most people produce up to three pints of it a day, and pass gas about 14 times a day, according to colon-rectal.com. This doesn't make it socially acceptable, however, and the discomfort makes it even less pleasant. The number-one remedy for flatulence in the entire essential oils apothecary is peppermint. In addition to the following remedy, you can get peppermint hard candy or other edible drops at any convenience store or drug store.

FLATULENCE PEPPERMINT RUB

Makes 1 treatment

4 to 6 drops peppermint essential oil

1. Place the peppermint essential oil in your palm and rub your hands together.
2. Then, rub your palms over your stomach and around your navel in a clockwise direction. The oil will be absorbed through your skin and will help relieve indigestion and flatulence.

Fluid Retention

Swollen feet, ankles, hands, wrists, or legs can come from a wide range of conditions. Perhaps you have a sedentary job, you like salty snacks, you're going through menopause, or you have one of many illnesses that can cause edema. Essential oils—accompanied by a diet lower in salt and daily exercise breaks—can help reduce the fluid and get your system functioning normally again.

FLUID RETENTION MASSAGE

Makes 3 treatments

4 tablespoons sweet almond oil or jojoba oil
10 drops each of any three of the following:
    carrot seed essential oil
    cypress essential oil
    fennel essential oil
    geranium essential oil
    grapefruit essential oil
    juniper essential oil
    rosemary essential oil

1. In a 4-ounce dark amber or cobalt glass bottle, mix the sweet almond oil with your 3 essential oils of choice (10 drops each).

2. Massage the area of fluid retention with this blend, using strokes that lead up or in toward the heart.

3. Repeat every 4 hours until the swelling subsides. Store the remaining blend in a cool place out of direct sunlight.

FOOTBATH FOR SWOLLEN ANKLES

Makes 1 treatment

2 drops cypress essential oil
2 drops frankincense essential oil
2 drops juniper essential oil

1. Fill a footbath tub with either warm or cool water, as you prefer.

2. Add the cypress, frankincense, and juniper essential oils.

3. Soak your feet for 10 to 15 minutes.

4. Repeat as desired until the swelling subsides.

Grief

Everyone experiences loss, and, for most of us, time and the comfort of friends and family are the only true remedies. Essential oils cannot take away the pain caused by the death of a loved one, and I would not be honest in telling you otherwise. They can, however, help you find balance and renewal when times seem hardest, by creating an atmosphere in which you can clear your head and see a way through the darkness. Use the calming, uplifting scents of sandalwood and myrrh for positive energy, and the exhilarating combination of citrus and spice to revitalize.

DIFFUSION FOR POSITIVE ENERGY

Makes 2 diffusions

2 drops bergamot essential oil
2 drops grapefruit essential oil
2 drops myrrh essential oil
2 drops sandalwood essential oil

1. In a small (5-mL) dark amber or cobalt glass bottle, mix the bergamot, grapefruit, myrrh, and sandalwood essential oils. Cap the bottle and shake well to combine.

2. Add 4 drops to your diffuser and turn it on.

3. Remain in the room for 15 to 30 minutes with the diffuser running.

4. Store the remaining blend in a cool place out of direct sunlight.

GRIEF RELIEF DIFFUSION

Makes 2 diffusions

2 drops bergamot essential oil
2 drops cinnamon essential oil
2 drops ginger essential oil
2 drops lemon essential oil
2 drops orange essential oil

continued >

1. In a small (5-mL) dark amber or cobalt glass bottle, mix the bergamot, cinnamon, ginger, lemon, and orange essential oils. Cap the bottle and shake well to combine.

2. Add 5 drops to your diffuser and turn it on.

3. Remain in the room for 15 to 30 minutes with the diffuser running.

4. Store the remaining blend in a cool place out of direct sunlight.

Hay Fever

More than 60 million people in the United States have hay fever, a fact that keeps the OTC pharmaceutical industry in business. Those medications can treat symptoms such as runny nose, clogged nasal passages, and streaming eyes, but they often come with side effects like dry mouth and grogginess. Try these natural essential oil treatments, with their antihistamine properties, instead.

HAY FEVER DIFFUSION

Makes enough for 2 hours of diffusion at 15 minutes per hour

2 drops anise essential oil
2 drops balsam fir essential oil
2 drops galbanum essential oil

1. Add the anise, balsam fir, and galbanum essential oils to your diffuser and turn it on.

2. Run the diffuser for 15 minutes every 2 hours.

3. You can also run your diffuser continually throughout the night by your bedside.

HAY FEVER SWAB

Makes 5 treatments

2 teaspoons olive oil
6 drops peppermint or spearmint essential oil
6 drops eucalyptus essential oil

1. In a small (15-mL) dark amber or cobalt glass bottle, mix the olive oil with the peppermint and eucalyptus essential oils.

2. With a cotton swab, dab a few drops of this blend around the outside of your nostrils.

3. Repeat as needed, especially if it wears away after you wipe your nose.

4. Do not use these oils without dilution in a carrier oil, as they can irritate the skin around your nostrils.

5. Store the remaining blend in a cool place out of direct sunlight.

Headache

In 1994, a study published in the journal *Cephalalgia* reported that peppermint oil combined with ethanol (alcohol) reduced pain sensitivity in human beings with headaches, achieving "a significant analgesic effect." This would have been no news to doctors in ancient Greece and Egypt, who had prescribed similar remedies for generations—but the study was good news to those who used essential oils in the twentieth century and beyond. Make the most of this effective remedy in your own essential oils practice.

HEADACHE SWAB

Makes 1 treatment

2 tablespoons vodka or grain alcohol
5 drops peppermint essential oil

1. In a small glass or metal bowl, mix the vodka with the peppermint essential oil.

2. Dip a cotton ball into the mixture and apply the liquid to your forehead, temples, and the back of your neck.

3. If you can, relax with your eyes closed until the pain subsides.

NOTE: If using grain alcohol, I recommend Everclear.

HEADACHE COLD COMPRESS

Makes 1 compress

1 cup cold water
5 drops peppermint essential oil

1. In a small glass or metal bowl, mix the water with the peppermint essential oil.
2. Place a washcloth on the surface of the water and let it become saturated.
3. Remove the cloth and wring it out until it no longer drips.
4. Lie down and place the cool washcloth on your forehead. Leave it there until it warms to room temperature.
5. Repeat this as needed to reduce headache pain.

Heartburn

When the acidic digestive juices in your stomach back up into your esophagus, you experience a discomfort known as heartburn—because of the burning sensation—or, in more modern parlance, acid reflux. Changes in your diet and an increase in exercise can help you manage this condition. As you get older, though, acid reflux can become a fact of life. If you'd like to try a natural remedy before turning to the many over-the-counter medications available for this issue, frankincense can have a calming effect on stomach and digestive issues. If, however, the heartburn does not subside after three days, see your doctor, as acid reflux can be a warning sign of a much more serious illness.

Makes 3 treatments

1 tablespoon olive oil
15 drops frankincense essential oil

1. In a 1-ounce dark amber or cobalt glass bottle, mix the olive oil with the frankincense essential oil. Cap the bottle and shake well to combine.
2. Before bed, rub 1 teaspoon of the blend on the stomach, throat, and chest.
3. Store the remaining blend in a cool place out of direct sunlight.

Hemorrhoids

Each hemorrhoid is a swollen vein in the anal canal, and can appear inside the canal or just outside the anus. They come from too much pressure—i.e., pushing—on the anal walls. Hemorrhoids feel much worse than they are, an important thing to remember when you're in considerable pain. Balsam, juniper, and frankincense essential oils help reduce swelling and calm the discomfort.

HEMORRHOID SITZ BATH

Makes 1 treatment

½ cup milk
3 drops balsam fir essential oil
3 drops juniper essential oil

1. Fill a bathtub with enough warm water to cover your hips.
2. Add the milk, along with the balsam fir and juniper essential oils. (The milk keeps the oils from floating on top of the water.)
3. Soak for 10 to 15 minutes, or until the water cools to body temperature.

Makes 1 treatment

2 drops frankincense essential oil

1. Cleanse the anal area with a moistened wipe.

2. Place the frankincense essential oil (neat) on a cotton ball.

3. Apply directly to the anal region.

4. Repeat after each bowel movement, after cleaning the area.

Hot Flashes

The changes in hormonal levels and activity that take place during menopause can throw a middle-aged woman's life into quiet chaos, and few things are more disruptive than the hot flashes that come on at any time of the day or night. Some essential oils can help balance hormones and modify or moderate this disturbing symptom, while others can offer cooling relief in the middle of the night.

HOT FLASH SPRITZ

Makes 10 to 15 treatments

6 tablespoons spring water
2 tablespoons witch hazel extract
8 drops peppermint essential oil
8 drops pine essential oil
8 drops Roman chamomile essential oil

1. In an 8-ounce glass or metal spray bottle, combine the water and witch hazel extract.

2. Add the peppermint, pine, and Roman chamomile essential oils. Cap the bottle and shake well to combine.

3. Spritz yourself with this blend when you feel a hot flash coming on. Store the remaining blend in a cool place out of direct sunlight, and remember to shake well before each use.

NEAT HOT FLASH HORMONE BALANCER

Makes 1 treatment

1 drop clary sage essential oil
1 drop geranium essential oil
1 drop peppermint essential oil

1. In the morning, apply 1 drop each (neat) of clary sage, geranium, and peppermint essential oils to the back of your neck.

2. Reapply later in the day, if needed.

HOT FLASH DIFFUSION

Makes 1 diffusion

3 drops clary sage essential oil

Add the clary sage essential oil to your diffuser and turn it on. Let it run overnight, or for 15 minutes of every hour that you're in the room during the day.

Indigestion

If you're on vacation, celebrating the holidays, or at a friend's home for dinner, you may find yourself with a sour stomach at the end of the evening. Indigestion can keep you up at night, and if it becomes chronic, your good times can take an unfortunate turn. Luckily, you have your personal apothecary to turn to when your digestive system isn't cooperating. Peppermint essential oil helps clear the head and settle the queasiness, and frankincense essential oil penetrates to aid digestion.

INDIGESTION RUB

Makes 1 treatment

1 teaspoon carrier oil of choice
4 or 5 drops of frankincense essential oil

continued >

1. Before bed, place the carrier oil in your palm. Add the frankincense essential oil to it.

2. Rub this blend on your stomach, throat, and chest.

INDIGESTION SCENTED PILLOW

Makes 5 to 10 treatments

2 tablespoons water
10 drops peppermint essential oil

1. In a 2-ounce glass or metal spray bottle, mix the water with the peppermint essential oil. Cap the bottle and shake well to combine.

2. Spritz your pillow lightly with this blend. The scent will promote relaxation and sleep even as it calms your stomach.

3. Store the remaining blend in a cool place out of direct sunlight.

Inflammation

A red, swollen joint can signal a significant injury or a painful arthritis flare-up. The sooner you treat the inflammation, the sooner real relief and healing can begin. Many essential oils have the ability to reduce the swelling, especially when paired with a cold compress, elevation, and rest.

INFLAMMATION COLD COMPRESS

Makes 1 compress

2 cups cold water
Ice cubes
2 drops balsam fir essential oil
2 drops frankincense essential oil
2 drops myrrh essential oil

1. In a medium glass or metal bowl, combine the water and ice cubes.
2. Add the balsam fir, frankincense, and myrrh essential oils.
3. Place a hand towel on the surface of the water and let it become saturated.
4. Lift the towel from the water and wring out the excess water.
5. Place the compress on the swollen area. Wrap it in plastic wrap to hold it in place and prevent dripping, but not so tightly that you cut off circulation.
6. Keep the compress on the swollen area until the towel warms to body temperature.
7. Repeat as needed until the swelling subsides.

INFLAMMATION WITH BRUISING COMPRESS

Makes 1 compress

2 cups cold water
Ice cubes
2 drops balsam fir essential oil
2 drops frankincense essential oil
2 drops helichrysum essential oil
2 drops myrrh essential oil

1. In a medium glass or metal bowl, combine the water and ice cubes.
2. Add the balsam fir, frankincense, helichrysum, and myrrh essential oils.
3. Place a hand towel on the surface of the water and let it become saturated.
4. Lift the towel from the water and wring out the excess water.
5. Place the compress on the bruised area. Wrap it in plastic wrap to hold it in place and prevent dripping, but not so tightly that you cut off circulation.
6. Keep the compress on the bruised area until the towel warms to body temperature.
7. Repeat as needed until the inflammation subsides.

Insomnia

There's nothing more maddening than not being able to sleep. Chronic insomnia can affect every aspect of your life, causing short-term memory impairment, irritability, an inability to concentrate, lapses in judgment, and even hallucinations. Aromatherapy can be key in getting your sleep cycle back on track, helping you overcome the barriers to sleep. Lavender has been proven in sleep studies in England and the United States to be especially helpful, improving sleep by as much as 20 percent. The scent of lavender essential oil slows the heart rate and lowers blood pressure, relaxing you so you can fall asleep.

INSOMNIA LAVENDER DIFFUSION

Makes 1 diffusion

3 drops lavender essential oil
3 drops Roman chamomile essential oil

1. Place the diffuser in your bedroom. Add the lavender and Roman chamomile essential oils to the diffuser and turn it on.

2. Let it run overnight.

3. Repeat every night to improve your sleep.

INSOMNIA-BUSTING BATH

Makes 1 bath

½ cup milk
3 drops lavender essential oil
2 drops Roman chamomile essential oil
1 drop benzoin (onycha) essential oil

1. In a small glass or metal bowl, mix the milk with the lavender, Roman chamomile, and benzoin essential oils.

2. Run a warm bath and then pour the blend into the warm water.

3. Enjoy the bath until it cools to body temperature.

4. Dry off and go to bed as soon after the bath as possible.

Itching

All kinds of issues can cause itching: dry weather, a new laundry detergent, mosquito bites, poison ivy, a fungal or yeast infection, or a food allergy. A number of essential oils can help, depending on the source of the itching: Tea tree and cypress oils are best for defeating yeast and fungus, cedarwood works against rashes, and pine can calm dry skin and an itchy scalp.

ITCH- AND FUNGUS-FIGHTING WASH

Makes 1 wash

½ cup warm water
2 drops cypress essential oil
2 drops tea tree essential oil

1. In a small glass or metal bowl, mix the water with the cypress and tea tree essential oils. Swish to combine.

2. Dip a clean washcloth into the blend and wash the affected area.

3. With a blow dryer set on low, dry the area completely.

4. Repeat as needed to combat the itching of athlete's foot or other fungal skin infections.

ITCHY DRY SKIN SOOTHER

Makes 12 treatments

¼ cup coconut oil
24 drops tea tree essential oil
12 drops cedarwood essential oil
12 drops pine essential oil

1. In a small glass or metal bowl, combine the coconut oil with the tea tree, cedarwood, and pine essential oils.

2. With your fingertips, smooth 1 teaspoon of the blend over the itchy skin.

3. Use twice daily—in the morning and before bed—to treat itching. Store the remaining blend in a 2-ounce dark amber or cobalt glass bottle or jar in a cool place out of direct sunlight.

Kitchen Care

Vinegar, water, and your favorite essential oil leave your home disinfected and smelling naturally clean, instead of irritating your nose with synthetic chemicals. Different essential oils kill different kinds of bacteria, so it's a good idea to choose a mix of five or six to cover the range of germs that may be at work in your kitchen or bathroom.

KITCHEN COUNTER WASH

Makes 1 application for a mid-size kitchen's counters
(make more if you have a large kitchen)

½ cup water
½ cup apple cider vinegar
4 drops cinnamon essential oil
4 drops eucalyptus essential oil
4 drops lavender essential oil
4 drops lemon essential oil
4 drops pine essential oil

1. In a medium glass or metal bowl or a small metal bucket, mix the water and apple cider vinegar with the cinnamon, eucalyptus, lavender, lemon, and pine essential oils.

2. Dip a clean sponge in the vinegar blend and wipe all your counters. Allow them to air dry.

3. Store any unused portion in a tightly sealed 8-ounce glass or metal spray bottle.

4. Use as often as your counters require it.

KITCHEN FLOOR CLEANER

Makes 1 application

1 gallon hot water
2 tablespoons unscented liquid castile soap
5 drops lemon essential oil
5 drops pine essential oil
5 drops tea tree essential oil

1. In a metal bucket, combine the water and castile soap with the lemon, pine, and tea tree essential oils.

2. Have ready a second bucket of hot water for rinsing the mop.

3. With a sponge mop, clean your floors with the water and oil blend, rinsing the mop in between in the bucket of plain water.

4. When you've finished washing the floor, empty and refill the bucket of plain water. Mop the floor again with the fresh plain water to rinse.

5. Allow the floor to air dry.

Labor and Delivery

If your physician, midwife, or doula agrees that using essential oils in the delivery room is safe for you and your baby, you may find that lavender, clary sage, and chamomile essential oils help you stay as calm and relaxed as possible. Mothers say that peppermint essential oil can help maintain energy while keeping you cool, and both lavender and frankincense can reduce the pain of contractions.

NOTE: Use peppermint with caution as it can be harmful to babies.

LABOR DIFFUSION

Makes 1 diffusion

3 drops chamomile (German or Roman) essential oil
3 drops lavender essential oil

1. Add the chamomile and lavender essential oils to your diffuser and turn it on.

2. Allow the diffuser to run for 15 minutes of every hour throughout labor and delivery.

LABOR ENERGY COMPRESS

Makes 1 treatment

½ cup cool water
3 drops peppermint essential oil

1. In a small glass or metal bowl, combine the water and peppermint essential oil.

2. Dip a washcloth into the cup and wet it thoroughly. Wring out the washcloth so it's damp but not dripping.

3. Place the cool cloth on the back of the neck of the woman in labor.

4. Remove the cloth when it no longer feels cool, or the mother no longer wants it.

5. *Stop using this when delivery is imminent, as peppermint can be harmful to babies.*

LABOR PAIN-RELIEF NEAT TREATMENT

Makes 1 treatment

2 or 3 drops frankincense essential oil

1. Place the frankincense drops (neat) on the area of the back where the pain is most acute. This may not substitute for an epidural, but it can take the edge off the worst of the pain.

2. Repeat as often as the medical professional or doula feels is safe.

Lactation

Depending upon how old your baby is, you may either be eager to produce more breast milk, or hoping to slow production so you can wean your child. Remedies for both are provided here. The secret to keeping breast milk production at optimal levels is fennel essential oil—it increases your milk by boosting estrogen production in your system. That said, you can have too much of a good thing by over-using fennel. Try it twice a day for a few days to see how it affects your lactation. If you're getting the results you want, take a break from it for a week or two to keep from overproducing and becoming engorged, or getting plugged ducts.

Peppermint essential oil is known to slow milk production, but some mothers find they have a sensitivity to it—and it can have an effect on the baby, as well. *Talk with your doctor before trying peppermint essential oil,* and dilute it well with a carrier oil before applying it to your skin. If you see redness, swelling, a rash, or hives, discontinue use immediately.

FENNEL RUB FOR LACTATION

Makes 4 treatments

½ cup avocado oil or coconut oil
8 drops fennel essential oil

1. In a 4-ounce dark amber or cobalt glass jar, combine the avocado oil and the fennel essential oil.
2. With your fingertips, apply the blend to your breasts and lymph area, avoiding the nipples.
3. Repeat this twice daily until you see an increase in milk production.
4. Discontinue use once you see the desired result. Wait 2 weeks before using again.
5. Store the remaining blend in a cool place out of direct sunlight.

NOTE: If you are concerned about overproduction, basil essential oil can be substituted for the fennel essential oil, and used for a longer period of time. It increases lactation, but may not produce the same abundant result.

BREAST MILK REDUCTION RUB

Makes 4 treatments

½ cup avocado oil or coconut oil
8 drops peppermint essential oil

1. In a 4-ounce dark amber or cobalt glass jar, combine the avocado oil with the peppermint essential oil.
2. With your fingertips, apply the mixture to your breasts and lymph area, avoiding the nipples.
3. Repeat this 3 times daily until you see a decrease in milk production.
4. Discontinue use once you see the desired result.
5. Store the remaining blend in a cool place out of direct sunlight.

SORE OR CRACKED NIPPLE RELIEF

Makes 1 treatment

1 teaspoon coconut oil
1 drop myrrh essential oil

1. On a spoon, combine the coconut oil with the myrrh essential oil.
2. With your fingertip, apply the blend to the nipple.
3. Repeat 2 to 3 times daily, as needed, after nursing.

Laundry Care

You don't need to spend a fortune on "green" laundry products to bring natural cleanliness to your family's clothing. Here, your essential oils add more scent than cleaning power, so mix and match your favorites to find the best combination for your laundry.

And skip the mysterious chemicals in commercial fabric softener products that soften our clothes; you can get the same effect from vinegar, baking soda, and lavender essential oil, and save some money, too.

POWDER LAUNDRY DETERGENT

Makes 72 loads

4 cups baking soda
3 cups washing soda
2 cups castile soap flakes (if solid, grated into a large glass or metal bowl)
3 to 4 drops lavender, lemon, or your favorite essential oil

1. In a large glass or metal bowl, stir together the baking soda, washing soda, castile soap, and lavender essential oil.

2. Store the powder in a large glass jar with a tight-fitting lid in a cool place out of direct sunlight.

3. Use 2 tablespoons per load of laundry for bright clothes with no artificial chemicals.

NATURAL FABRIC SOFTENER

Makes 1 load

1/2 cup white vinegar
2 tablespoons baking soda
1/2 teaspoon (50 drops) lavender essential oil

1. In a small glass or metal bowl, stir together the vinegar and baking soda until the baking soda dissolves.

2. Add the lavender essential oil.

3. Pour this blend into the rinse cycle (or the fabric-softener compartment) while your clothes are washing.

Lice

Head lice are common among children from every background, in every school, in every part of the country, and are highly contagious between children who play or go to school together. When your child has head lice, your first priority is to get those bugs gone. You will have to change your child's morning schedule to include removing the lice and preventing them from multiplying. Slow the lice down to make them easier to remove with a lice comb, and take preventive measures to keep them from reappearing. Here are some methods that work.

INITIAL LICE TREATMENT

Makes 1 treatment

¼ to ⅓ cup olive oil or sweet almond oil
White vinegar, for soaking

1. Coat your child's hair with the olive oil. Essential oils won't help at this point.

2. With a hair comb, separate the hair into sections. Use hair clips to fasten the hair out of the way so you can work on one section at a time.

3. With a lice comb, comb through your child's hair to find the lice. Remove them with the comb and discard them.

4. Wash your child's hair using her regular shampoo. Rinse and repeat.

5. Dry your child's hair with a towel. Launder the towel immediately.

6. Soak the lice comb and any other tools you used in vinegar for 30 minutes.

7. Repeat this process daily for 1 week. After the first week, continue to comb through your child's hair with the lice comb for another 2 weeks to be sure the lice are gone.

OVERNIGHT LICE TREATMENT

Makes 7 treatments

¼ cup olive oil
15 to 20 drops of one of the following:
    anise essential oil
    cinnamon essential oil
    clove essential oil
    eucalyptus essential oil
    lavender essential oil
    tea tree essential oil

1. In a small glass or metal bowl, mix the olive oil with the essential oil of choice.

2. With a cotton ball, apply this blend to your child's scalp.

3. Leave it on at least 12 hours (overnight).

4. In the morning, comb through your child's hair with a lice comb, and shampoo as usual.

5. Store the remaining blend in a cool place out of direct sunlight.

ALCOHOL SPRAY FOR LICE PREVENTION

Makes 14 treatments (enough for 2 weeks)

½ cup rubbing alcohol
15 to 20 drops of one of the following (use the same essential oil
    you selected for Overnight Lice Treatment):
        anise essential oil
        cinnamon essential oil
        clove essential oil
        eucalyptus essential oil
        lavender essential oil
        tea tree essential oil

1. In an 8-ounce glass or metal spray bottle, mix the alcohol with the essential oil of choice. Cap the bottle and shake well to combine.

continued >

2. Daily for 2 weeks, spray the blend on your child's hair before bed.

3. Use the lice comb to remove any remaining lice and to check for reappearance.

4. Store the remaining blend in a cool place out of direct sunlight.

Menstrual Issues

If you want to relieve the pain of menstrual cramps but don't want the caffeine and diuretics found in OTC PMS pills, try these simple remedies. Not only are they natural, but they also have a sound basis in recent scientific research: A 2011 study published in 2012 in the journal *Evidence-Based Complementary and Alternative Medicine* found that aromatherapy massage using clary sage, marjoram, cinnamon, ginger, and geranium essential oils in sweet almond oil was more effective at reducing the pain of menstrual cramps than acetaminophen (Tylenol). A 2013 study published by the same source determined that cinnamon, clove, lavender, and rose essential oils delivered by massage also slowed excessive bleeding during menses.

MENSTRUAL MASSAGE OIL

Makes 1 treatment

1 teaspoon sweet almond oil
2 drops cinnamon essential oil
2 drops clary sage essential oil
2 drops geranium essential oil
2 drops ginger essential oil
2 drops marjoram essential oil

1. In a spoon, blend the sweet almond oil with the cinnamon, clary sage, geranium, ginger, and marjoram essential oils.

2. With your fingertips, rub this blend into your abdomen and lower back.

3. Repeat twice daily to relieve the pain of menstrual cramps.

HEAVY-BLEEDING MENSTRUAL RELIEF

Makes 1 treatment

1 teaspoon sweet almond oil
2 drops cinnamon essential oil
2 drops clove essential oil
1 drop lavender essential oil
1 drop rose essential oil

1. In a spoon, mix the sweet almond oil with the cinnamon, clove, lavender, and rose essential oils.

2. With your fingertips, rub this blend into your abdomen and lower back.

3. Repeat twice daily to relieve the pain of menstrual cramps and ease the heavy bleeding.

MENSTRUAL PAIN WARM COMPRESS

Makes 1 compress

½ cup warm water
2 drops cinnamon essential oil
2 drops clove essential oil
1 drop lavender essential oil
1 drop rose essential oil

1. In a small glass or metal bowl, mix the water with the cinnamon, clove, lavender, and rose essential oils.

2. Place a washcloth on the surface of the water and let it become saturated.

3. Remove the cloth from the water and wring out the excess water.

4. Place the wet compress on your abdomen.

5. Remove the compress when it cools to the point that it no longer feels warm.

6. Repeat twice daily as needed for pain and heavy menstrual bleeding.

Migraine

Migraines are a specific kind of headache that can cause problems with vision and light sensitivity, nausea, and, in severe cases, even vomiting. Regulating body temperature when the early symptoms appear can help migraine sufferers stop a headache from forming by returning the body's blood flow to normal. Cayenne essential oil, available from most companies, functions as an anti-inflammatory aid and helps relax the blood vessels and soothe the pain.

MIGRAINE PREVENTION THROUGH WARM HANDS

Makes 1 treatment

1 quart warm water (about 110°F)
5 drops ginger essential oil
5 drops lavender essential oil

1. In a quart-size glass or metal bowl, combine the water with the ginger and lavender essential oils.
2. At the first sign of a migraine, soak your hands in this blend for at least 3 minutes.

WARM COMPRESS FOR MIGRAINES

Makes 1 compress

½ cup warm water
5 drops ginger essential oil
5 drops lavender essential oil

1. In a small glass or metal bowl, combine the water with the ginger and lavender essential oils.
2. Place a washcloth on the surface of the water and let it become saturated.
3. Remove the cloth from the water and wring out the excess water.
4. Place the warm compress on your forehead.

5. Remove the compress when it cools to the point that it no longer feels warm.

6. Repeat as needed for pain.

NOTE: Warmth helps here to regulate body temperature and dilate the blood vessels.

CAYENNE CREAM FOR MIGRAINE

Makes 1 treatment

1 tablespoon unscented hand cream or lotion
5 drops cayenne essential oil

1. In your palm, blend the hand cream and cayenne essential oil.

2. Smooth this onto your forehead and temples.

3. Repeat once an hour until the pain subsides.

NOTE: Never use neat cayenne essential oil directly on your skin, as it can be very irritating.

Muscle Pain and Aches

If you increase your physical activity on weekends or you've just started a new exercise regimen, chances are you get muscle aches. These blends—paired with ice or a cold compress—can reduce inflammation and ease the pain. In addition, basil and juniper essential oils can provide penetrating relief from pain.

MUSCLE PAIN COLD COMPRESS

Makes 1 compress

2 cups cold water
3 drops myrrh essential oil
2 drops balsam fir essential oil
2 drops pine essential oil

continued >

1. In a medium glass or metal bowl, mix the water with the myrrh, balsam fir, and pine essential oils.

2. Place a hand towel on the surface of the water and let it become saturated.

3. Remove the towel, wring out the excess water, and place it on the aching muscle.

4. Wrap it with plastic wrap to hold it in place and keep it from dripping, but not so tightly that you cut off circulation.

5. Leave the compress in place until it warms to room temperature.

MUSCLE ACHE MASSAGE

Makes 4 treatments

4 teaspoons sweet almond oil
4 drops lavender essential oil
4 drops rosemary essential oil
2 drops ginger essential oil

1. In a 1-ounce dark amber or cobalt glass bottle, mix the sweet almond oil with the lavender, rosemary, and ginger essential oils. Cap the bottle and shake well to combine.

2. Massage your aching muscle with a few drops of this blend.

3. Use every few hours until the ache subsides.

4. Store the remaining blend in a cool place out of direct sunlight until your next use.

MUSCLE PAIN MASSAGE

Makes 4 treatments

4 teaspoons jojoba oil
4 drops black pepper essential oil
4 drops cinnamon essential oil
2 drops ginger essential oil

1. In a 1-ounce dark amber or cobalt glass bottle, mix the jojoba oil with the black pepper, cinnamon, and ginger essential oils. Cap the bottle and shake well to combine.

2. Massage your painful muscles with a few drops of this blend.

3. Store the remaining blend in a cool place out of direct sunlight until your next use.

Muscle Spasms

Quite a number of things can cause cramps in your legs and feet that wake you in the middle of the night: tired, overtaxed muscles; a magnesium or calcium deficiency; or lowered electrolytes from dehydration. When you leap out of bed in pain and limp around the room until the knot goes away, it's good to have your essential oil blend ready to rub on the spot, easing the pain and allowing you to go back to sleep.

QUICK MASSAGE FOR MUSCLE SPASMS

Keep this blend by your bedside for soothing relief.

Makes 3 to 5 treatments

1 tablespoon sweet almond oil
1 tablespoon basil essential oil
1 tablespoon juniper essential oil

1. In a 2-ounce dark amber or cobalt glass bottle, mix the sweet almond oil with the basil and juniper essential oils. Cap the bottle and shake well to combine.

2. When a cramp strikes, pour a few drops of this blend into your palm and rub it into the skin over the cramped muscle until it relaxes.

3. Store the remaining blend in a cool place out of direct sunlight.

CHARLEY HORSE TREATMENT

Makes 3 to 5 treatments

1 tablespoon sweet almond oil
1 tablespoon basil essential oil
1 tablespoon juniper essential oil

1. In a 2-ounce dark amber or cobalt glass bottle, mix the sweet almond oil with the basil and juniper essential oils. Cap the bottle and shake well to combine.
2. Rub a few drops of this blend into the cramped muscle 3 times daily to relieve pain and restore flexibility.
3. After each rub, apply a warm compress or a hot pack to help the oils absorb into your skin, and to loosen the sore muscle.
4. Store the remaining blend in a cool place out of direct sunlight.

Nail Care

All kinds of daily hazards make fingernails thin and brittle: washing dishes, using nail-polish remover, dry air, and the normal wear and tear of using our hands. Essential oils and a number of carrier oils can fight these conditions and help you develop stronger, thicker, more attractive nails.

Essential oils can help fight fungus that can appear on even the most well-groomed toenails, as well. OTC medications can stop the fungus eventually, but many people pay podiatrists a small fortune to debride the thickened material that results. If you are determined and deliberate, you can defeat toenail fungus with essential oils.

STIMULATING CUTICLE RUB

Makes 5 to 7 treatments

1½ tablespoons jojoba oil
2 drops lavender essential oil
1 drop myrrh essential oil
1 drop peppermint essential oil

1. In a 1-ounce dark amber or cobalt glass bottle, mix the jojoba oil with the lavender, myrrh, and peppermint essential oils.

2. Each night before bed, rub the mixture into your cuticles.

3. Keep the excess by your bedside, tightly sealed, to remind yourself to use it.

TOENAIL FUNGUS SWAB

Makes 12 treatments

¼ cup jojoba oil or coconut oil
12 drops mustard essential oil
12 drops spikenard essential oil
12 drops tea tree essential oil

1. In a 4-ounce dark amber or cobalt glass bottle, mix the jojoba oil with the mustard, spikenard, and tea tree essential oils.

2. Saturate a cotton ball in 1 teaspoon of the blend.

3. Place the cotton ball on the affected nail (use several cotton balls if more than one nail is affected) and hold there for 10 minutes.

4. Do this at least twice daily, in the morning and evening, until the fungus is gone. (This may take several weeks.)

5. Store the remaining blend in a cool place out of direct sunlight.

NAIL-CARE FOOT SOAK

Makes 1 treatment

1 cup apple cider vinegar
10 drops cinnamon essential oil
10 drops balsam fir essential oil
10 drops tea tree essential oil

1. Fill a footbath or basin with warm water. Add the apple cider vinegar along with the cinnamon, balsam fir, and tea tree essential oils.

2. Soak your feet for 20 to 30 minutes. Dry thoroughly with a clean towel.

3. Do this at least twice daily until the fungus clears.

Nasal Congestion

When your head feels like it's stuffed with cotton and you're struggling to get air through your nasal passages, there's nothing like eucalyptus to penetrate that blockage. Eucalyptus essential oil provides the strongest concentration of eucalyptus on the market, so it takes just a few drops to reduce the swelling in nasal passages and restore your ability to breathe. Lemon, clove, and peppermint essential oils all have their own penetrating properties, so a bath with several of these will do wonders for the unpleasant effects of a cold.

NASAL CONGESTION VAPOR RUB

Makes 1 treatment

1 teaspoon carrier oil of choice
3 drops rosemary essential oil
2 drops eucalyptus essential oil
1 drop lemon essential oil

1. In your palm, combine the carrier oil with the rosemary, eucalyptus, and lemon essential oils.
2. Gently rub this blend on your chest, neck, cheekbones, and around your nose, following the line of your sinus cavities.

NASAL DECONGESTION BATH

Makes 1 treatment

2 drops each of any combination of the following:
    clove essential oil
    eucalyptus essential oil
    lavender essential oil
    lemon essential oil
    peppermint essential oil
    tea tree essential oil

1. Run a warm bath and add your essential oils of choice.
2. Settle into the bath, breathe the scents, and relax until the water cools.

Makes 1 diffusion

3 drops eucalyptus essential oil

1. Add the eucalyptus essential oil to your diffuser and turn it on.
2. Let the diffuser run all night in your bedroom as you sleep. The penetrating vapors will reduce your nasal congestion and help you get a good night's rest.

Nausea and Vomiting

Whether you are suffering from a stomach virus, food poisoning, the symptoms of colitis, or the rigors of chemotherapy, there's no worse feeling than being nauseated. You may not want to think about swallowing, but you still need to breathe, so try these soothing remedies. Lying still, either in bed or in a warm bath, can help you unclench muscles and get soothing relief for your digestive tract. If you are vomiting, patchouli essential oil is the best possible remedy for your plight.

NAUSEA-CALMING DIFFUSION

Makes enough for 3 to 4 hours of diffusion at 15 minutes per hour

2 drops basil essential oil
2 drops bergamot essential oil
2 drops German chamomile essential oil

1. Add the basil, bergamot, and German chamomile essential oils to your diffuser and turn it on.
2. Run the diffuser for 15 minutes out of every hour until your nausea subsides.

STOMACH-SETTLING BATH

Makes 1 treatment

3 drops cassia essential oil
3 drops spearmint essential oil

1. Run a warm bath.

2. Add the cassia and spearmint essential oils.

3. Inhale deeply as you relax in the bath.

VOMITING REMEDY

Makes 12 to 15 treatments

1 tablespoon jojoba oil
12 drops patchouli essential oil

1. In a small (15-mL) dark amber or cobalt glass bottle, mix the jojoba oil and patchouli essential oil. Cap the bottle and shake well to combine.

2. Massage 3 drops of this blend over your navel and behind your ears.

3. Place a warm compress over your stomach after you apply the oil, then lie back and relax.

4. Store the remaining blend in a cool place out of direct sunlight.

NOTE: Inhaling the scent of patchouli oil neat on a cotton ball every 10 to 15 minutes can also help relax the muscles and reduce the contractions that come with vomiting.

Oily Hair and Scalp

All too often, we reach for expensive chemicals in upscale salon products to deal with simple issues such as oily hair, when what we really need are nature-made solutions. This combination of glycerin and herbal-scented essential oils will leave your hair shiny and luxurious, instead of stripping out what's natural and replacing it with factory formulas.

Makes 12 treatments

¾ cup water
¾ cup white vinegar
1½ teaspoons vegetable glycerin
6 drops bay laurel essential oil
6 drops cedarwood essential oil
6 drops lemon essential oil

1. In a 16-ounce dark amber or cobalt glass bottle, mix the water, vinegar, and glycerin with the bay laurel, cedarwood, and lemon essential oils. Cap the bottle and shake well to combine.

2. Wash your hair as usual and rinse it well.

3. Pour a small amount of the conditioner into your hand. Work it into your hair and comb it through. Wait 1 minute and rinse, or, for best results, leave it in your hair.

4. Store the remaining blend in a cool place out of direct sunlight.

Oily Skin

You may be surprised at the number of essential oils that can help you tame the sheen on your skin. A powerful acne fighter, tea tree essential oil is nonetheless mild enough to use directly on your skin without diluting it. Rosemary adds astringent and antibacterial properties that fight acne as well as oily skin. Many other essential oils lend their astringent qualities to your daily cleansing, helping control the return of the sheen by balancing the pH levels in your skin. Using grapeseed oil in blends adds another level of astringent. Think how you'll feel when the shine on your face comes just from within.

1:1 SWAB FOR OILY SKIN

Makes 1 treatment

3 drops grapeseed oil
3 drops of any one of the following:

bergamot essential oil
clary sage essential oil
cypress essential oil
frankincense essential oil
geranium essential oil
helichrysum essential oil
lavender essential oil
lemon essential oil
lemongrass essential oil

orange essential oil
patchouli essential oil
peppermint essential oil
Roman chamomile
  essential oil
rosemary essential oil
sandalwood essential oil
tea tree essential oil
ylang-ylang essential oil

1. On a cotton ball, combine the grapeseed oil and your essential oil of choice.

2. Smooth the blend over your clean face.

3. Do this once daily after you wash your face.

TEA TREE AND ROSEMARY SWAB FOR OILY SKIN

Makes 1 treatment

2 drops tea tree essential oil
1 drop rosemary essential oil

1. On a cotton ball, combine the tea tree and rosemary essential oils.

2. Smooth this over your face to refresh your skin after a workout or before going out.

OILY SKIN MASK

Makes enough mask base for 4 to 5 treatments

For the mask base
2 ounces green clay (powder)
1 tablespoon corn flour

1 tablespoon mask base
1 tablespoon brewer's yeast
1 tablespoon water
1 drop juniper essential oil
1 drop lavender essential oil

1. In a 4-ounce jar, make the mask base by mixing the green clay and corn flour.

2. In a small glass or metal bowl, make the mask by mixing the mask base, brewer's yeast, and water with the juniper and lavender essential oils. Stir to combine.

3. Apply to your clean face.

4. Leave it on for 15 minutes, then rinse and pat dry.

5. Save the remaining mask base to mix for future applications.

Perspiration

If you're one of the many people who sweat more than others, you already know that you can't cover your body with antiperspirant and expect to continue your day in comfort. Commercial preparations work fine under your arms, but using them liberally everywhere else curbs your body's natural process of cooling itself. Instead, this natural remedy may help slow the flow. Not only will you see less surface perspiration, but you will also smell like a botanical garden.

ROLL-ON BODY ANTIPERSPIRANT

Makes 2 ounces

2 tablespoons grapeseed oil
48 drops lavender essential oil
36 drops clary sage essential oil
24 drops cypress essential oil

continued >

1. In a 2-ounce bottle with a roll-on applicator top, combine the grapeseed oil with the lavender, clary sage, and cypress essential oils.

2. After your daily shower, roll this blend on areas of excessive sweating.

3. Store the remaining blend in a cool place out of direct sunlight.

Pet Care

In general, the jury is still out about the use of essential oils with pets. Animals often have a greater sensitivity to scents than humans do, so they may be attracted or repelled by scented oils. If you do try aromatherapy or medicinal use of oils around your pets, be sure to leave them an escape route if they don't react well to the scent. Keep in mind that dogs and cats will lick any area of their skin or fur treated with an essential oil, so they will ingest the solution—making the use risky, even if the essential oil is well-diluted in an ingestible carrier oil.

Animals react differently to essential oils than we do, because they metabolize substances differently from humans. Before you begin to diffuse essential oils in your home, talk to your veterinarian about signs you should watch for to judge how your pet is responding (well, badly, or not at all) to the new substance in the air.

Pets can react well at the start and develop allergic reactions later. Cats are particularly sensitive to essential oils, so you may want to forego their use entirely in areas frequented by your cat. Some essential oils can cause liver or kidney toxicity in sensitive animals, including cats, so avoid "hot" oils including birch, cassia, cinnamon, clove, mustard, oregano, thyme, and wintergreen in homes with a cat. Cats also should not receive any topical use of tea tree oil.

Until science catches up, people with pets need to be selective about their use of essential oils in diffusers, vaporizers, or sprays that may linger in rooms frequented by animals, and in the oils used on a pet's skin or hair. Above all, don't add essential oils to your animal's water or food, as the oils don't break up in water and your pet will consume them in their most concentrated—and dangerous—form.

Postpartum Depression

When a new mother's negative emotions after her baby is born dominate the positive ones, the mother has postpartum depression. This potentially debilitating condition can be compounded by sleep deprivation and a crying baby, making the situation seem more dire with each day. Postpartum depression is a medical condition requiring a doctor's care, not a "phase," and the fact that nursing mothers can't take antidepressants makes it that much harder to cope with its realities. Essential oils offer a natural means of coping with postpartum depression. Bergamot and clary sage essential oils help lift the spirit, while frankincense essential oil calms the nerves and takes the edge off a tense situation.

POSTPARTUM DIFFUSION

Makes enough for 3 to 4 hours of diffusion at 15 minutes per hour

2 drops bergamot essential oil
2 drops clary sage essential oil
2 drops frankincense essential oil

1. Add the bergamot, clary sage, and frankincense essential oils to your diffuser and turn it on.

2. In your bedroom or other room where you can spend some time alone, or with family, use the diffuser for 15 minutes per hour.

NOTE: Talk to your pediatrician before bringing your newborn baby into the room when the diffuser is running.

FRAGRANT POSTPARTUM MASSAGE

Makes 1 treatment

1 teaspoon sweet almond oil
1 teaspoon (100 drops) clary sage essential oil

continued >

1. In a small glass cup, combine the sweet almond oil with the clary sage essential oil.

2. Apply this blend to your hips, thighs, upper arms, and other areas of dense tissue, where your body stores your hormones.

3. Apply daily to restore balance and elevate your mood as your body recovers from the tumult of pregnancy and childbirth.

POSTPARTUM INHALATION

Makes 1 treatment

1 or 2 drops of one of the following:
Bergamot essential oil
Clary sage essential oil
Frankincense essential oil

1. Place 1 or 2 drops of the essential oil on a tissue.

2. Carry the tissue in a pocket, and inhale a whiff whenever you have a moment.

Prostate Issues

When the prostate cells do not get enough nutrients and fresh, healthy blood to move toxins out of the prostate, prostatitis develops. The toxins come from the nearby colon, a diet low in fruits and vegetables, and a lack of exercise—all things that lead to a wide range of health problems. Prostatitis causes pain and inflammation, difficulty with urination, and lower back pain. Left untreated, it can lead to larger health issues.

Essential oils are not a substitute for a healthy diet and daily exercise, but catching the infection before it becomes acute can help get the prostate back on the right track. Make the following remedies part of a healthy regimen that renews your overall well-being. If you don't see improvement within a few days, seek medical attention to rule out the possibility of prostate cancer.

PROSTATE SITZ BATH

Makes 1 treatment

2 tablespoons milk
3 drops sandalwood essential oil

1. Run a warm bath, deep enough to cover your hips.

2. In a small glass or metal bowl, mix the milk with the sandalwood essential oil, and then pour this into the bath.

3. Sit in the bath and relax until the water cools to room temperature.

4. Repeat daily until your symptoms improve. If symptoms do not improve within 3 days, consult your physician.

LOWER BACK MASSAGE FOR PROSTATE ISSUES

Makes 6 treatments

1 tablespoon sweet almond oil
1½ teaspoons Roman chamomile essential oil
1½ teaspoons sandalwood essential oil

1. In a 2-ounce dark amber or cobalt glass bottle, mix the sweet almond oil with the Roman chamomile and sandalwood essential oils. Cap the bottle and shake well to combine.

2. Massage 1 teaspoon of the blend into your lower back and abdomen to relieve pain and tension.

3. Repeat twice daily until the condition improves. Store the remaining blend in a cool place out of direct sunlight.

Psoriasis

A skin disorder in which new skin cells are produced faster than the normal rate, psoriasis is more common than you may realize. The skin develops patches of new skin that are covered with old, dead skin flakes, resulting in a condition as uncomfortable as it is unsightly. Virtually any change in routine can trigger an episode—a stressful or emotional time, an illness or infection, or a major life event. Smoking, excessive alcohol use, and even cold weather can be enough to make psoriasis reappear.

Essential oils can help with the symptoms, but like the pharmaceutical solutions currently available, they cannot bring about a swift resolution to the problem. Rose essential oil is particularly effective in calming skin irritation, making it a first choice for many psoriasis sufferers. Juniper essential oil stimulates circulation, bringing healing to the inflamed patches of skin, and helichrysum essential oil eases inflammation while it promotes healing. Don't give up after two or three treatments; patience and diligence can help you see results from the use of essential oils.

PSORIASIS APPLICATION

Makes 12 treatments

¼ cup avocado oil or jojoba oil
36 drops juniper essential oil
36 drops patchouli essential oil
24 drops cistus essential oil
24 drops tea tree essential oil

1. In a 4-ounce dark amber or cobalt glass jar, combine the avocado oil with the juniper, patchouli, cistus, and tea tree essential oils. Cover the jar and shake to mix.

2. Apply this blend directly to your affected skin.

3. Use twice daily. If this treatment irritates your skin or aggravates the condition, discontinue use immediately. Store the remaining blend in a cool place out of direct sunlight.

PSORIASIS INFLAMMATION-REDUCER

Makes 12 treatments

¼ cup jojoba oil or avocado oil
24 drops helichrysum essential oil
24 drops rose essential oil

1. In a 4-ounce dark amber or cobalt glass bottle, mix the jojoba oil with the helichrysum and rose essential oils. Cap the bottle and shake well to combine.

2. Apply 1 teaspoon of the blend directly on any inflamed areas to calm the redness and swelling.

3. Do this twice daily until the inflammation subsides. Store the remaining blend in a cool place out of direct sunlight.

Rashes

Many factors can cause a rash—a food allergy, sensitivity to a new detergent or soap, excessive sweating, a hot day, physical contact with certain plants, a fungal infection, and a wide range of less common triggers. Pairing the right essential oils with the cause of your rash can be tricky, especially if you have no idea how you got the itchy bumps or hives. The following recipes will calm the itching and give you quick relief from the worst of the condition.

One rash can be worse than all others: poison ivy, the result of an oil called urushiol, to which more than 90 percent of people are allergic. Urushiol transfers itself from the poison ivy plant to your shoes, clothing, backpack, and anything else you may be carrying, and then onto your skin. Getting rid of this pernicious and persistent oil takes multiple washings with strong, oil-cutting soap. Dawn dish detergent is a good one for this. Most people don't know they've brushed against the plant, however, so when the rash appears, be ready with any of the five essential oils that have anti-itch properties: lavender, peppermint, Roman chamomile, rose, and wintergreen. In addition, tea tree oil has been known to have a soothing effect specifically on reactions to poison ivy.

RASH-FIGHTING TOPICAL APPLICATION

Makes 3 treatments

1 tablespoon avocado oil
1 tablespoon of any one of the following:
  lavender essential oil
  peppermint essential oil
  Roman chamomile essential oil
  rose essential oil
  wintergreen essential oil

1. In a 2-ounce dark amber or cobalt glass bottle, mix the avocado oil with the essential oil of choice.

2. Apply this directly to the itchy rash.

3. Repeat as often as necessary to combat the itching. Store the remaining blend in a cool place out of direct sunlight.

POISON IVY NEAT APPLICATION

Makes 1 treatment

6 drops tea tree essential oil

1. Pour the tea tree essential oil directly on a cotton ball and apply it to the rash.

2. Repeat as often as needed to quell the itching until the rash clears up.

RASH AND HIVES ANTI-ITCH PASTE

Makes 8 treatments

2 cups water
3 tablespoons baking soda
5 drops chamomile (German or Roman) essential oil
2 drops peppermint essential oil
3 tablespoons bentonite clay

1. In a medium glass or metal bowl, mix the water and baking soda with the chamomile and peppermint essential oils.

2. In a small metal bowl, combine the bentonite clay with ¼ cup of the essential oil and water solution. Stir to mix.

3. Apply the paste directly to the rash. Allow it to stay on for 45 minutes and then wash it off.

4. Repeat as needed to calm the itching.

Respiratory Infection

When a cold or sinus infection descends into your chest, it can cause coughing, difficulty breathing, shortness of breath, and the feeling that there's a weight pressing against your chest. You can break up the congestion using tried-and-true eucalyptus essential oil and peppermint essential oil, the same ones that have found their way into a number of OTC products such as vapor rubs and cough drops.

RESPIRATORY INFECTION CHEST RUB

Makes 4 treatments

¼ cup sweet almond oil
20 drops eucalyptus essential oil
5 drops basil essential oil
5 drops cedarwood essential oil
5 drops peppermint essential oil

1. In a small glass or metal bowl, mix the sweet almond oil with the eucalyptus, basil, cedarwood, and peppermint essential oils.

2. Stir to combine.

3. Rub 1 tablespoon of this blend on your chest to loosen congestion. Repeat 3 to 4 times daily, as needed.

4. Store the remaining blend in a cool place out of direct sunlight.

Makes enough for 8 to 10 hours of diffusion at 10 to 15 minutes per hour

20 drops eucalyptus essential oil
20 drops lavender essential oil
5 drops peppermint essential oil

1. In a small (5-mL) dark amber or cobalt glass bottle, mix the eucalyptus, lavender, and peppermint essential oils. Cap the bottle and shake well to combine.

2. Add a few drops of this blend to a diffuser, turn it on, and run it in your room for 10 to 15 minutes every hour.

3. Store the remaining blend in a cool place out of direct sunlight.

Scars

Scars from an injury, surgery, chicken pox, or acne can take a long time to heal, and an even longer time to fade. You may treat your scar for as long as six months before it is fully healed, so it's a good idea to mix your lotions and oils in batches, enough for a week or more at a time.

Geranium essential oil has an unusual ability to revitalize skin and encourage rapid healing, and sandalwood essential oil is known for its ability to boost the body's natural immunity. When combined with the healing properties of the other essential oils in these remedies, they can help speed the recovery process.

SCAR LOTION

Makes 12 treatments

¼ cup coconut oil
36 drops geranium essential oil
36 drops cedarwood essential oil

1. In a 4-ounce dark amber or cobalt glass bottle, mix the coconut oil with the geranium and cedarwood essential oils. Cap the bottle and shake well to combine.

2. With your fingertips, apply 1 teaspoon of the blend to your scar twice daily. Continue until the scar has healed and faded (this may take months).

3. Store the remaining blend in a cool place out of direct sunlight.

SCAR OIL TREATMENT

Makes 10 treatments

3 tablespoons sweet almond oil or avocado oil
¼ teaspoon vitamin E oil
1 teaspoon cistus essential oil
30 drops frankincense essential oil
30 drops juniper essential oil
30 drops myrrh essential oil
30 drops sandalwood essential oil

1. In a 4-ounce dark amber or cobalt glass bottle, mix the sweet almond oil, vitamin E oil, and the cistus, frankincense, juniper, myrrh, and sandalwood essential oils.

2. Pour an amount about the size of a nickel into your palm. (Use more if the scar is large or if there are multiple scars.)

3. Apply twice daily to the scar. It will take time for the scar to fade, so continue treatment for as long as required.

4. Store the remaining blend in a cool place out of direct sunlight.

Sexual Desire

A substance is considered an aphrodisiac if it stimulates passion and sexual arousal, which means that as many as 60 different essential oils can qualify as aphrodisiacs. While no substance on earth will magically arouse someone who does not want to be aroused, some essential oils can help create an environment and a mood for sexual desire. Anything that reduces stress and anxiety, improves mood, and creates sensual awareness can open the door to sexual desire.

CUSTOM BLEND TO SET THE MOOD

To create your own blend for sexual arousal, choose a range of essential oils from a number of different groups. Pick three or four scents to blend at the most; too many create a cloud of indistinct aromas that can work against your amorous plans. Consider:

- **Citrus essential oils** for sweetness, to take the edge off spicier oils: grapefruit, lemon, lime, neroli, petitgrain, orange, mandarin, and tangerine.

- **Spice essential oils** for musky scents: allspice, anise, black pepper, cardamom, cinnamon, clove, coriander, frankincense, ginger, myrrh, and nutmeg.

- **Mint essential oils** for a bright, crisp note: peppermint, spearmint, or horse mint.

- **Conifer essential oils** for the hint of wilderness that may be particularly effective for the rugged adventurer (or your lumberjack fantasy!): balsam fir, cedarwood, cypress, fir needle, pine, Scotch pine, or spruce.

- **Exotic essential oils** for a sense of far-off lands: fennel, patchouli, sandalwood, star anise, vanilla, and vetiver.

- **Floral essential oils** for the light notes of romance: bergamot, geranium, jasmine, lavender, Roman chamomile, rose, and ylang-ylang.

AROUSAL DIFFUSION

Makes 1 diffusion

1. Choosing from the list on page 186, add 1 or 2 drops each of your chosen essential oils to your diffuser, and turn it on.

2. Run the diffuser at 15-minute intervals, or allow it to run continuously.

SENSUAL MASSAGE

Makes 1 to 2 treatments

2 tablespoons sweet almond oil or jojoba oil
6 to 8 drops each of up to 3 oils from the list on page 186.

1. In a 2-ounce dark amber or cobalt glass bottle, mix the sweet almond oil with the 3 essential oils of choice.

2. Before use, cap the bottle and shake well to combine. Store the remaining blend in a cool place out of direct sunlight.

Sinusitis

Whether you have a cold or a chronic sinus condition, pressure and blockage in your nasal passages can lead to a sinus infection, which can spread to become an ear infection or drop down to cause bronchitis. The best way to avoid this is to keep your sinuses clear, and there's nothing like steam and the penetrating effect of essential oils to open up your head. Tea tree essential oil in any steam blend can clear your sinuses while infusing them with natural germ-killing antiseptic.

SINUSITIS STEAM TREATMENT

Makes 1 treatment

2 cups steaming-hot water
5 drops tea tree essential oil
3 drops eucalyptus or pine essential oil

continued >

1. Fill a medium glass or metal bowl with the steaming water. Add the tea tree and eucalyptus essential oils.

2. Place a trivet or hot pad on a surface you can bend your head over. Place the bowl on the trivet. Cover your head with a towel and bend over the steaming water, using the towel to trap the steam. Breathe deeply.

3. Come up for fresh air when you need it, and continue to breathe the steam until the water cools.

4. Repeat as often as needed to keep your sinuses clear.

Skin Infections

When you spot strange red bumps that fill up with pus or burst and form a crust on the skin, a bacterial infection, such as cellulitis or impetigo, may be at work. This begins with a cut or scrape that breaks the skin, especially in children who may continue to play and get dirt and germs in the untended cut, leading to a nasty infection.

Essential oils can give relief at the topical level and help clear up the pimple-like lesions as quickly as possible. The root of these infections comes from strep or staph bacteria, and both can be dangerous when left untreated. See your doctor for antibiotics (especially if the infection shows up on your child), and finish the prescription to cure the infection completely.

SKIN INFECTION SWAB

Makes 3 treatments

1 tablespoon jojoba oil or coconut oil
3 drops frankincense essential oil
3 drops lavender essential oil
3 drops tea tree essential oil

1. In a 1-ounce dark amber or cobalt glass bottle, mix the jojoba oil with the frankincense, lavender, and tea tree essential oils. Cap the bottle and shake well to combine.

2. Soak a cotton ball in the oil blend and then swab the affected area. Do this 3 times daily until the infection subsides.

3. Store the remaining blend in a cool place out of direct sunlight.

Stiff Neck

Did you sleep "wrong" and wake up with a stiff neck? Or did your neck pain develop at work on a particularly stressful day? The essential oils you use to combat the pain will differ depending on the reason for your stiffness. Peppermint and lavender, two of the most versatile essential oils, will provide penetrating relief while promoting relaxation. Basil essential oil will help reduce swelling in a pulled muscle, relieving neck pain and easing stiffness.

LAVENDER AND PEPPERMINT NECK RUB

Makes 1 treatment

1 teaspoon sweet almond oil
2 drops lavender essential oil
2 drops peppermint essential oil

1. In your palm, mix the sweet almond oil with the lavender and peppermint essential oils.

2. Rub (or have someone rub) this blend into the stiff muscles at the base of your neck and along your shoulders.

3. Repeat twice daily as needed to relieve stiffness.

INFLAMMATION-INDUCED STIFF NECK RUB

Makes 1 treatment

1 teaspoon avocado oil or jojoba oil
2 drops basil essential oil

1. In your palm, mix the avocado oil with the basil essential oil.

2. Rub (or have someone rub) this blend on the stiff part of the neck and corresponding shoulder muscles.

3. Repeat twice daily until the stiffness subsides.

Makes 1 treatment

1 teaspoon olive oil
2 drops cypress essential oil
2 drops peppermint essential oil

1. In your palm, mix the olive oil with the cypress and peppermint essential oils.

2. Rub (or have someone rub) this blend on the stiff part of the neck and corresponding shoulder muscles.

3. Repeat twice daily until the stiffness subsides.

Stress

Throughout this chapter, you'll find essential oil solutions and treatments for a considerable range of stress symptoms: headache, muscle aches and pains, indigestion, stiff neck, and insomnia, for example. Your essential oils can address all these ailments, as well as the feelings of stress that cause this discomfort. Aromatherapy in massage, a relaxing bath, a diffusion, or a quick whiff right out of the bottle can provide the release you need to overcome stress and face the next challenge.

STRESS-RELIEVING MASSAGE

Makes 3 to 4 treatments

¼ cup sweet almond oil
10 drops lavender essential oil
6 drops Roman chamomile essential oil
4 drops sandalwood essential oil
4 drops ylang-ylang essential oil
1 drop benzoin (onycha) essential oil

1. In a 4-ounce dark amber or cobalt glass bottle, combine the sweet almond oil with the lavender, Roman chamomile, sandalwood, ylang-ylang, and benzoin essential oils. Cap the bottle until needed.

2. Shake the blend and massage at day's end to release stress before bed. Store the remaining blend in a cool place out of direct sunlight.

STRESS-REDUCTION BATH

Makes 5 baths

20 drops lavender essential oil
12 drops Roman chamomile essential oil
8 drops sandalwood essential oil
8 drops ylang-ylang essential oil
2 drops benzoin (onycha) essential oil
½ cup milk

1. In a small (5-mL) dark amber or cobalt glass bottle, mix the lavender, Roman chamomile, sandalwood, ylang-ylang, and benzoin essential oils. Cap the bottle and shake to combine.

2. In a small glass or metal bowl, stir together the milk and 10 drops of the oil blend. Cap the bottle with the remaining oil to use for your next stressful day.

3. Run a warm bath and, while the water is running, add the milk-oil mixture to the bath to disperse it into the water.

4. Relax in the tub for 15 minutes, or until the water cools to body temperature.

5. Store the remaining blend in a cool place out of direct sunlight.

STRESS-LOWERING SPRAY

Makes 2 ounces

¼ cup water
6 drops frankincense essential oil
6 drops juniper essential oil
4 drops anise essential oil
4 drops sandalwood essential oil
1 drop benzoin essential oil

continued >

1. In a 4-ounce glass or metal spray bottle, mix the water with the frankincense, juniper, anise, sandalwood, and benzoin essential oils. Cap the bottle and shake well to combine.

2. Spritz this blend in any room in your home, as often as you like. Breathe and de-stress. Store the remaining blend in a cool place out of direct sunlight.

Thinning Hair

Everyone loses about 20 to 100 strands of hair per day, but if your hairline is traveling up your forehead or your hair has lost its full body, natural remedies can help slow the process. Essential oils combined with massage can stimulate your scalp and improve circulation, bringing good health to your hair follicles. Not only can they help you retain more hair, but they also restore your hair's natural luster, rescuing it from commercial conditioners, gels, mousses, and other products. Get rid of any hair products that contain high levels of detergents, phosphates, artificial scents, alkalizing substances, and wax and choose an unscented natural shampoo from your favorite natural food store. Essential oils will help you achieve the desired result, especially when combined with jojoba oil, one of nature's best conditioners.

HAIR LOSS MINIMIZING MASSAGE

Makes 5 to 10 treatments

½ cup jojoba oil
20 drops cedarwood essential oil
20 drops lavender essential oil
20 drops rosemary essential oil
20 drops thyme essential oil

1. In a 8-ounce dark amber or cobalt glass bottle, mix the jojoba oil with the cedarwood, lavender, rosemary, and thyme essential oils.

2. Wash your hair as usual.

3. In your palm, pour an amount of the conditioner blend about the size of a quarter. Massage your scalp with this blend for 1 minute, then rinse.

4. Use every other day to minimize hair loss.

5. Store the remaining blend in a cool place out of direct sunlight.

NATURAL SHAMPOO FOR THINNING HAIR

Makes 8 to 10 treatments

20 drops bay laurel essential oil
20 drops clary sage or ylang-ylang essential oil
20 drops cypress or juniper essential oil
1 (4-ounce) bottle natural shampoo, such as Dr. Bronner's
or Kiehl's

1. Add the bay laurel, clary sage, and cypress essential oils to the bottle of shampoo. Cap the bottle and shake well to combine.

2. Use this blend every time you wash your hair. Store the remaining blend in a cool place out of direct sunlight.

NOTE: Unless you work up a sweat at the gym every day, there's no need to wash your hair daily. Washing every other day or twice a week will keep your scalp and hair from drying out and becoming brittle.

Urinary Tract Infection

UTIs, inflammation of the bladder caused by bacteria, cause a wide range of discomforts ranging from the constant sensation that you have to urinate, to feeling like you're climbing the walls when you use the bathroom. They can even alter behavior and cause hallucinations, especially in the elderly. Using essential oils at the first sign of irritation can prevent a full infection, and bergamot's antibacterial properties will help kill the bacteria causing the irritation, quelling the infection before it sets in.

In addition to this treatment, drinking a glass of plain water or cranberry juice every hour will also help your symptoms.

Makes 8 to 10 treatments

1 cup water
30 drops bergamot essential oil

1. In a small pot over high heat, combine the water and bergamot essential oil. Bring the water to a boil, remove from the heat, and let it cool completely.

2. Dip a clean cotton ball in this blend and swab the urethra area with the water.

3. Store the water in a sterile container, and use every 2 hours during the day until the symptoms subside. If you are still symptomatic after 2 days, consult your doctor.

4. Store the remaining blend in a cool place out of direct sunlight.

Varicose Veins

Another name for broken blood vessels—clusters of red, blue, or purple vein lines on your legs—is varicose veins. When the vessel breaks, the blood pools in your leg, pressing on the vein walls and making them weaker. They start to twist and become visible, and you see them as varicose veins. The good news is they do not have to be permanent; with some diligence and perseverance you can help them heal and disappear.

Helichrysum essential oil is the gold standard for this, but it can be expensive, and cypress will do the job as effectively. Cypress essential oil is highly effective against varicose veins because it promotes circulation and strengthens the capillary walls in your blood vessels.

VARICOSE VEINS MOISTURIZER

Makes 1 treatment

6 drops of extra-virgin olive oil
3 drops bergamot essential oil
3 drops ylang-ylang essential oil

1. In your palm, combine the olive oil with the bergamot and ylang-ylang essential oils.
2. Rub your palms together 3 times in a circular motion to blend the oils.
3. Smooth this blend onto the affected area 2 to 3 times daily, starting below the veins and moving upward toward your heart. Massage for about 2 minutes.

VARICOSE VEINS COLD COMPRESS

Makes 1 compress

2 cups cold water
10 drops helichrysum essential oil
10 drops cistus essential oil

1. In a medium glass or metal bowl, mix the water with the helichrysum and cistus essential oils.
2. Place a washcloth on the surface of the water and let it become saturated.
3. Remove the cloth and wring until it is damp but not dripping.
4. Apply the compress to the varicose veins. Wrap it in plastic wrap to hold the compress in place, but not so tightly that it cuts off circulation.
5. Leave the compress in place for 10 to 15 minutes—it's best to elevate your leg for this.
6. Apply the compress to the affected area 2 to 3 times daily.

Makes 4 to 6 treatments

2 tablespoons olive oil
25 drops cypress essential oil

1. In a 2-ounce dark amber or cobalt glass bottle, mix the olive oil with the cypress essential oil. Cap the bottle and shake well to combine.
2. With your fingertips, massage 1 teaspoon of the blend to the area above the broken blood vessel. Do not massage below the blood vessel, as that puts more pressure on the capillary and could prolong the healing process.
3. Do this twice daily.
4. Store the remaining blend in a cool place out of direct sunlight.

Vertigo

If you see the room tilt and feel motion when you're standing still, you may be experiencing vertigo. This is caused by particles in your inner ear that have become lodged in place, blocking the normal flow of fluids that maintain your balance. You can often arrest an attack of vertigo by changing the position of your head and dislodging the particles, allowing them to move freely again. If you're lying down, though, and watching the room spin, a little peppermint essential oil will help you feel grounded again.

NEAT TOPICAL PEPPERMINT FOR VERTIGO

Makes 1 treatment

4 to 6 drops peppermint essential oil

1. Apply 1 drop of peppermint essential oil directly from the bottle to your forehead, the back of your neck, and behind your ears to help clear your head. Breathe.

2. Repeat this after 10 minutes if the vertigo does not pass.

3. If you still have vertigo after the second treatment, consider contacting your physician.

Whooping Cough

Modern medicine has a proven vaccine to prevent your child from getting whooping cough, but, if your child has not had the vaccine, he might contract this illness. The coughing comes in fits that make the child gasp for air, scaring your child and you until the spasm has passed. See a doctor when your child has whooping cough, and get the prescription medication that will cure this illness. Use essential oils only as complementary remedies to calm the coughing spasms, loosen congestion, and promote wellness.

WHOOPING COUGH CHEST RUB

Makes 5 treatments

¼ cup sweet almond oil
20 drops eucalyptus essential oil
5 drops basil essential oil
5 drops cedarwood essential oil
5 drops peppermint essential oil

1. In a small glass or metal bowl, combine the sweet almond oil with the eucalyptus, basil, cedarwood, and peppermint essential oils. Stir to mix.

2. Rub this blend on the child's chest to loosen congestion.

3. Store the remaining blend in a cool place out of direct sunlight.

NOTE: *Do not use this treatment on children younger than 2 years old,* as the eucalyptus and peppermint oils can cause a spasm in their throat muscles, closing off the airway.

Makes enough for 3 hours of diffusion at 10 to 15 minutes per hour

20 drops eucalyptus essential oil
20 drops lavender essential oil

1. In a small (5-mL) dark amber or cobalt glass bottle, mix the eucalyptus and lavender essential oils.
2. Add a few drops of this blend to a diffuser and turn it on.
3. Run the diffuser in your child's room for 10 to 15 minutes every 3 hours.
4. Store the remaining blend in a cool place out of direct sunlight.

Wounds

Every cut or wound has the potential to allow pathogens—the organisms that cause infection and sepsis—to enter the body. Once you have stopped the bleeding by applying pressure to the wound, clean the wound with plain water and an antiseptic. Examine it to determine how severe the damage is.

Essential oils can help protect the site from infection. Lavender and tea tree essential oils are two of the best essential oils for warding off infection and sepsis. German and Roman chamomile, clary sage, helichrysum, myrrh, and myrtle all reduce inflammation. If you have calendula oil on hand, use it as the carrier oil. It has been shown to stimulate cell growth and promote healing, but in an emergency situation, olive oil is a perfectly sensible oil to use.

WOUND HEALING OINTMENT

Makes 3 treatments

2 tablespoons calendula oil or olive oil
10 drops lavender essential oil
5 drops myrrh essential oil
5 drops tea tree essential oil

1. In a 2-ounce dark amber or cobalt glass bottle, mix the calendula oil with the lavender, myrrh, and tea tree essential oils. Cap the bottle and shake well to combine.

2. Use sterile gauze or a cotton swab to apply this blend to cover the wound.

3. Bandage the wound with a sterile gauze pad and tape it firmly in place to keep it covered.

4. Store the remaining blend in a cool place out of direct sunlight.

Glossary

adaptogen: A substance that helps us adapt to environmental factors that cause stress, and reduces the potential for damage by this stress.

analgesic: Provides pain relief.

anesthetic: Induces relaxation and sleep.

anoint: To pour oil over an object or a person to consecrate it in the eyes of God.

antibacterial: Kills bacteria, which can cause infections.

antifungal: Inhibits the growth of fungus.

antigalactogogue: Reduces the flow of breast milk.

anti-inflammatory: Reduces redness and swelling.

antimicrobial: Kills microorganisms such as bacteria and fungus.

antirheumatic: Relieves pain and stiffness in the extremities and back.

antiseptic: Protects against sepsis and septic infection.

antispasmodic: Relieves muscle spasms.

antiviral: Counteracts viruses.

aphrodisiac: Stimulates interest in sex.

aromatic application method: Using steam, vapor, or diffusion to propel an essential oil into the air for therapeutic benefit.

astringent: Tightens skin and removes oiliness.

carrier oil: An oil used to dilute and "carry" the essential oil to the skin or other application.

circulatory: Improves blood circulation.

decongestant: Reduces mucus congestion in the head and chest.

digestive: Promotes digestion and relieves a sour stomach.

disinfectant: Guards against infection.

diuretic: Counteracts water retention.

emmenagogue: Promotes menstrual flow.

expectorant: Assists in loosening phlegm.

febrifuge: Reduces fever.

fungicide: Kills fungal infections.

ingestion: Swallowing an essential oil.

insecticide: Wards off and kills insects.

irritant: Produces an inflammatory response.

laxative: Promotes bowel movements.

neat: Using an essential oil full strength on the skin, a cotton ball, or a tissue.

photodynamic: The property of some essential oils' molecules that make skin more susceptible to the sun's ultraviolet (UV) rays. These oils react to UV light and cause sunburn, which is why this reaction is called *phototoxicity* or *photosensitivity*.

probiotic: Adds live bacteria.

pure: A marketing term that implies the content of a bottle is 100 percent essential oil.

relaxant: Encourages muscles to relax.

sedative: Aids in relaxation and sleep.

sensitization: Making the skin more sensitive to sunlight and, therefore, more in danger of harmful effects (e.g., cancer) from exposure to it. A number of essential oils can cause sensitization if used full strength.

stimulant: Quickens functional activity.

sudorific: Causes perspiration.

terpenes: Also known as hydrocarbons, terpenes are the molecules within a plant that give the plant its unique scent.

therapeutic grade: A marketing term meant to imply that an essential oil has met a standard set by the government for purity. No such standards exist.

tonic: Strengthens and invigorates.

topical application method: Using essential oils by applying them to the skin after diluting them in a carrier oil.

tranquilizer: Causes sleep.

vermifuge: Expels parasites.

volatile organic compounds (VOCs): Naturally occurring substances in essential oils that have a beneficial effect on the mind and body.

Oils in Scripture
Book, Chapter, Verse

ALOES

Numbers 24:6
Psalms 45:8
Proverbs 7:17
Song of Solomon 4:14
John 19:39

ANISE

Matthew 23:23

BALM

Genesis 37:25, 43:11
Jeremiah 8:22, 46:11, 51:8
Ezekiel 27:17

BAY

Psalms 37:35

BDELLIUM

Genesis 2:12
Numbers 11:7

CALAMUS

Exodus 30:23
Song of Solomon 4:14
Ezekiel 27:19

CAMPHIRE

Song of Solomon 1:14, 4:13

CASSIA

Exodus 30:24
Psalms 45:8
Ezekiel 27:19

CEDAR

Leviticus 14:4, 14:6, 14:49, 14:51, 14:52
Numbers 19:6, 24:6
Judges 9:15
2 Samuel 5:11, 7:2, 7:7
1 Kings 4:33, 5:6, 5:8, 5:10, 6:9, 6:10, 6:15, 6:16, 6:18, 6:20, 6:36, 7:2, 7:3, 7:7, 7:11, 7:12, 9:11, 10:27
2 Kings 14:9
1 Chronicles 14:1, 17:1, 17:6, 22:4
2 Chronicles 1:15, 2:3, 2:8, 9:27, 25:18
Ezra 3:7
Job 40:17
Psalms 29:5, 80:10, 92:12, 104:16, 148:9
Song of Solomon 1:17, 5:15, 8:9
Isaiah 2:13, 9:10, 14:8, 37:24, 41:19, 44:14
Jeremiah 22:7, 22:14, 22:15, 22:23
Ezekiel 17:3, 17:22, 17:23, 27:5, 27:24, 31:3, 31:8
Amos 2:9
Zephaniah 2:14
Zechariah 11:1, 11:2

CINNAMON

Exodus 30:23
Proverbs 7:17
Song of Solomon 4:14
Revelation 18:13

CORIANDER

Exodus 16:31
Numbers 11:7

CUMIN

Isaiah 28:25, 28:27
Matthew 23:23

CYPRESS

Isaiah 44:14

FIR

2 Samuel 6:5
1 Kings 5:8, 5:10, 6:15, 6:34, 9:11
2 Chronicles 2:8, 3:5
Psalms 104:17
Song of Solomon 1:17
Isaiah 14:8, 37:24, 41:19–20, 55:13, 60:13
Ezekiel 31:8
Hosea 14:8
Nahum 2:3
Zechariah 11:12

FRANKINCENSE

Exodus 30:34
Leviticus 2:1 2:2, 2:15, 2:16, 5:11, 6:15, 24:7
Numbers 5:15
1 Chronicles 9:29
Nehemiah 13:5, 13:9
Song of Solomon 3:6, 4:6, 4:14
Matthew 2:11
Revelation 18:13

GALBANUM

Exodus 30:34

HYSSOP

Exodus 12:22
Leviticus 14:4, 14:6, 14:49,
   14:51, 14:52
Numbers 19:6, 19:18
1 Kings 4:33
Psalms 51:7
John 19:29
Hebrews 9:19

JUNIPER

1 Kings 19:4–5
Job 30:4
Psalms 120:4

MINT

Matthew 23:23
Luke 11:42

MUSTARD SEED

Matthew 13:31–32, 17:20
Mark 4:31
Luke 13:19, 17:6

MYRRH

Genesis 37:25, 43:11
Exodus 30:23
Esther 2:12
Psalms 45:8
Proverbs 7:17
Song of Solomon 1:13, 3:6, 4:6,
   4:14, 5:1, 5:5, 5:13
Matthew 2:11
Mark 15:23
John 19:39

MYRTLE

Nehemiah 8:15
Isaiah 41:19, 55:13
Zechariah 1:8, 1:10, 1:11

ONYCHA

Exodus 30:34

PINE

Nehemiah 8:15
Isaiah 41:19, 60:13

ROSE OF SHARON

Song of Solomon 2:1

RUE

Luke 11:42

SAFFRON

Song of Solomon 4:14

SHITTAH/SHITTIM

Exodus 25:5, 25:10, 25:13, 25:23,
25:28, 26:15, 26:26, 26:37,
27:1, 27:6, 30:1, 30:5, 35:7,
35:24, 36:20, 36:31, 36:36,
37:1, 37:4, 37:10, 37:15, 37:25,
37:28, 38:1, 38:6
Deuteronomy 10:3
Isaiah 41:19

SPIKENARD

Song of Solomon 1:12, 4:13, 4:14
Mark 14:3
John 12:3

WORMWOOD

Deuteronomy 29:18
Proverbs 5:4
Jeremiah 9:15, 23:15
Lamentations 3:15, 3:19
Amos 5:7
Revelation 8:11

Ailments and Oils
Quick Reference Guide

AILMENT	SUGGESTED ESSENTIAL OILS	METHOD OF APPLICATION
Acne	Carrot seed Juniper Orange Roman chamomile Tea tree	Swab
Aging skin	Geranium Myrrh Sandalwood	Massage Rub
Air freshener	Eucalyptus Pine Tea tree	Spray
Anger	Balsam fir or Fir needle Clary sage Galbanum German chamomile Lavender Peppermint Roman chamomile Rose Sandalwood	Diffusion Spray

AILMENT	SUGGESTED ESSENTIAL OILS	METHOD OF APPLICATION
Anxiety	Cedarwood	Bath
	Geranium	Spray
	Lavender	
	Sandalwood	
	Spearmint	
	Ylang-ylang	
Arthritis	Balsam fir or	Rub
	Fir needle	
	Clove	
	Eucalyptus	
	Sandalwood	
	Spearmint	
Asthma	Eucalyptus	Steam
	Frankincense	Vapor rub
	Geranium	
	Lavender	
	Peppermint	
Back pain	Balsam poplar	Rub
	Cassia	Soak
	Clary sage	
	Eucalyptus	
	Lavender	
	Rosemary	
Bathroom care	Grapefruit	Scrub
	Lavender	Spray
	Lemon	
	Tea tree	
Blisters	Benzoin	Neat drop
	Frankincense	Swab
	German chamomile	
	Lavender	
	Myrtle	

AILMENT	SUGGESTED ESSENTIAL OILS	METHOD OF APPLICATION
Bloating	Coriander Lemon Peppermint	Rub
Body odor	Cassie Cistus Cumin Eucalyptus Geranium Lavender Lemon Lime Peppermint Pine Spearmint Tea tree Thyme	Roll-on Spray Stick
Bronchitis	Eucalyptus Rosemary	Diffusion Steam
Bug bites and stings	Galbanum German chamomile Lavender Peppermint Roman chamomile Wintergreen	Compress Neat
Bug repellent	Cedarwood Citronella Eucalyptus Geranium Ginger Lavender Lemongrass Vetiver	Skin application Spray

AILMENT	SUGGESTED ESSENTIAL OILS	METHOD OF APPLICATION
Cellulite	Cypress Fennel Grapefruit Helichrysum Juniper Lemon Rosemary Sage	Massage
Chapped lips	Cistus Frankincense Myrrh	Gel Lip balm
Chilblains	Cedarwood Helichrysum Lavender Myrrh Sandalwood	Bath Layering
Colds and flu	Balsam fir or Fir needle Eucalyptus Lavender Lemon Myrrh Rosemary Tea tree	Steam Vapor rub
Colic	Geranium Lavender	Massage Warm compress
Conjunctivitis	Rose	Warm compress

AILMENT	SUGGESTED ESSENTIAL OILS	METHOD OF APPLICATION
Cough	Balsam fir or Fir needle	Vaporizer Vapor rub
	Eucalyptus	
	Frankincense	
	German chamomile	
	Ginger	
	Lavender	
	Oregano	
	Roman chamomile	
	Sandalwood	
	Tea tree	
Cradle cap	Geranium	Massage
	Rose geranium	
Cuts and scrapes	Eucalyptus	Neat
	Lavender	Wash
	Lemon	
	Pine	
	Sandalwood	
	Spikenard	
	Tea tree	
Diaper rash	Lavender	Skin application
	Yarrow	Wash
Diarrhea	Cedarwood	Massage
	Eucalyptus	
	Lavender	
	Tea tree	
Ear infection	Cedarwood	Cotton ball
	Lavender	Swab
	Roman chamomile	
	Rosemary	
Eczema	Frankincense	Skin application
	Geranium	
	Helichrysum	
	Thyme	

AILMENT	SUGGESTED ESSENTIAL OILS	METHOD OF APPLICATION
Fatigue	Anise	Diffusion
	Bdellium	Spray
	Cassia	
	Cinnamon	
	Frankincense	
	Lemon	
	Peppermint	
	Pine	
Fever	Eucalyptus	Cold compress
	Peppermint	Neat
	Spearmint	
Flatulence	Peppermint	Rub
Fluid retention	Carrot seed	Footbath
	Cypress	Massage
	Fennel	
	Frankincense	
	Geranium	
	Grapefruit	
	Juniper	
	Rosemary	
Grief	Bergamot	Diffusion
	Cinnamon	
	Ginger	
	Grapefruit	
	Lemon	
	Myrrh	
	Orange	
	Sandalwood	
Hay fever	Anise	Diffusion
	Balsam fir or	Swab
	Fir needle	
	Eucalyptus	
	Galbanum	
	Peppermint	
	Spearmint	

AILMENT	SUGGESTED ESSENTIAL OILS	METHOD OF APPLICATION
Headache	Peppermint	Cold compress
		Swab
Heartburn	Frankincense	Rub
Hemorrhoids	Balsam fir	Bath
	Frankincense	Swab
	Juniper	
Hot flashes	Clary sage	Diffusion
	Geranium	Neat
	Peppermint	Spray
	Pine	
	Roman chamomile	
Indigestion	Frankincense	Rub
	Peppermint	Spray
Inflammation	Balsam fir	Cold compress
	Frankincense	
	Helichrysum	
	Myrrh	
Insomnia	Benzoin	Bath
	Lavender	Diffusion
	Roman chamomile	
Itching	Cedarwood	Skin application
	Cypress	Wash
	Pine	
	Tea tree	
Kitchen care	Cinnamon	Wash
	Eucalyptus	
	Lavender	
	Lemon	
	Pine	
	Tea tree	
Labor and delivery	Chamomile	Cold compress
	Frankincense	Diffusion
	Lavender	Neat
	Peppermint	

AILMENT	SUGGESTED ESSENTIAL OILS	METHOD OF APPLICATION
Lactation production	Fennel Myrrh Peppermint	Rub Skin application
Laundry care	Lavender Lemon	Liquid Powder
Lice	Anise Cinnamon Clove Eucalyptus Lavender Tea tree	Scalp application Spray
Menstrual issues	Cinnamon Clary sage Clove Geranium Ginger Lavender Marjoram Rose	Massage Rub Warm compress
Migraine	Cayenne Ginger Lavender	Skin application Soak Warm compress
Muscle pain and aches	Balsam fir or Fir needle Black pepper Cinnamon Ginger Lavender Myrrh Pine Rosemary	Cold compress Massage
Muscle spasms	Basil Juniper	Massage

AILMENT	SUGGESTED ESSENTIAL OILS	METHOD OF APPLICATION
Nail care	Balsam fir	Rub
	Cinnamon	Soak
	Lavender	Swab
	Myrrh	
	Peppermint	
	Spikenard	
	Tea tree	
Nasal congestion	Clove	Bath
	Eucalyptus	Rub
	Lavender	
	Lemon	
	Peppermint	
	Rosemary	
	Tea tree	
Nausea and vomiting	Basil	Bath
	Bergamot	Diffusion
	Cassia	Massage
	German chamomile	
	Patchouli	
	Spearmint	
Oily hair and scalp	Bay laurel	Conditioner
	Cedarwood	
	Lemon	

AILMENT	SUGGESTED ESSENTIAL OILS	METHOD OF APPLICATION
Oily skin	Bergamot	Mask
	Clary sage	Swab
	Cypress	
	Frankincense	
	Geranium	
	Helichrysum	
	Juniper	
	Lavender	
	Lemon	
	Lemongrass	
	Orange	
	Patchouli	
	Peppermint	
	Roman chamomile	
	Rosemary	
	Sandalwood	
	Tea tree	
	Ylang-ylang	
Perspiration (excessive)	Clary sage	Roll-on
	Cypress	
	Lavender	
Postpartum depression	Bergamot	Diffusion
	Clary sage	Massage
	Frankincense	Neat
Prostate issues	Roman chamomile	Bath
	Sandalwood	Massage
Psoriasis	Cistus	Neat
	Helichrysum	Skin application
	Juniper	
	Patchouli	
	Rose	
	Tea tree	

AILMENT	SUGGESTED ESSENTIAL OILS	METHOD OF APPLICATION
Rashes	German chamomile	Neat
	Lavender	Paste
	Peppermint	Skin application
	Roman chamomile	
	Rose	
	Tea tree	
	Wintergreen	
Respiratory infection	Basil	Diffusion
	Cedarwood	Rub
	Eucalyptus	
	Lavender	
	Peppermint	
Scars	Cedarwood	Topical application
	Cistus	
	Frankincense	
	Geranium	
	Juniper	
	Myrrh	
	Sandalwood	
Sexual desire	More than 40 choices (see page 186)	Diffusion Massage
Sinusitis	Eucalyptus	Steam
	Pine	
	Tea tree	
Skin infections	Frankincense	Swab
	Lavender	
	Tea tree	
Stiff neck	Basil	Rub
	Cypress	
	Lavender	
	Peppermint	

AILMENT	SUGGESTED ESSENTIAL OILS	METHOD OF APPLICATION
Stress	Anise Benzoin Frankincense Juniper Lavender Roman chamomile Sandalwood Ylang-ylang	Bath Massage Spray
Thinning hair	Bay laurel Cedarwood Clary sage Cypress Juniper Lavender Rosemary Thyme Ylang-ylang	Massage Shampoo
Urinary tract infection	Bergamot	Swab
Varicose veins	Bergamot Cistus Cypress Helichrysum Ylang-ylang	Cold compress Massage Topical application
Vertigo	Peppermint	Neat
Whooping cough	Basil Cedarwood Eucalyptus Lavender Peppermint	Diffusion Vapor rub
Wounds	Lavender Myrrh Tea tree	Topical application

References

Adams, Case. "Essential Oils Treat Menses Pain and Excessive Bleeding." Heal Naturally. Accessed April 4, 2016. www.realnatural.org/menstruation-pain-and-excessive-bleeding-treated-with-essential-oil-massage/.

Althea Press. *Essential Oils for Beginners*. Berkeley, CA: Althea Press, 2013.

——. *Essential Oils Natural Remedies*. Berkeley, CA: Althea Press, 2015.

AromaHut Institute. "Onycha Essential Oil." Accessed March 17 & 23, 2016. www.healwithoil.com/onycha-essential-oil/.

——. "Saffron Essential Oil." Accessed March 25, 2016. www.healwithoil.com/saffron-essential-oil/.

AromaWeb. "Anise Essential Oil." Accessed March 17, 2016. www.aromaweb.com/essential-oils/anise-oil.asp.

——. "Aromatherapy and Aphrodisiacs." Accessed June 24, 2014. www.aromaweb.com/articles/aromatherapyaphrodisiacs.asp.

——. "Aromatherapy Recipes to Help Energize and Stay Alert." Accessed June 22, 2014. www.aromaweb.com/recipes/energize.asp.

——. "Bay Laurel Essential Oil." Accessed March 19, 2016. www.aromaweb.com/essential-oils/bay-laurel-oil.asp.

——. "Cassia Bark Essential Oil." Accessed March 20, 2016. www.aromaweb.com/essential-oils/cassia-oil.asp.

——. "Fir Needle Essential Oil." Accessed March 22, 2016. www.aromaweb.com/essential-oils/fir-needle-oil.asp.

——. "Myrrh Essential Oil." Accessed March 23, 2016. www.aromaweb.com/essential-oils/myrrh-oil.asp.

Artisan Aromatics. "Balsam Poplar Essential Oil." Accessed March 17, 2016. https://artisanessentialoils.com/shop/all-essential-oils/balsam-poplar-essential-oil/.

Aura Cacia. "Sandalwood Essential Oil." Accessed March 17, 2016. www.auracacia. com/auracacia/aclearn/features/sandalwood.html.

Benencia, F., and M. C. Courrèges. "Antiviral Activity of Sandalwood Oil against Herpes Simplex Viruses -1 and -2." Phytomedicine 6, no. 2 (May 1999): 191–23. Accessed March 29, 2016. www.ncbi.nlm.nih.gov/pubmed/10374251.

Bible Hub. "Isaiah 41." Accessed March 25, 2016. http://biblehub.com /commentaries/barnes/isaiah/41.htm.

———. "Song of Solomon 2:1." Accessed March 24, 2016. http://biblehub.com /songs/2-1.htm.

Bible.org. "Where Did the Idea that Jesus is the Rose of Sharon Come From?" Accessed March 24, 2016. http://bible.org/question/where-did-idea-jesus -rose-sharon-come.

BibleStudyTools.com. "Oil." Baker's Evangelical Dictionary of Biblical Theology. Accessed March 28, 2016. www.biblestudytools.com/dictionary/oil/.

Bratcher, Dennis. "A New Day Dawns: Verse Commentary on Isaiah 60:1–3, 15–22." The Voice: Biblical and Theological Resources for Growing Christians. Accessed March 24, 2016. www.crivoice.org/isa60.html.

Callahan, Jeff. "Top 10 Essential Oils for Sleep & Insomnia." EssentialOilBenefits. org. Accessed June 23, 2014. http://essentialoilbenefits.org/top-10-essential -oils-sleep-insomnia.

Camp Wander (blog). "Breast Feeding & Essential Oils." March 23, 2014. http://campwander.com/2014/03/breast-feeding-essential-oils/.

ChristianAnswers.net. "Onycha." WebBible Encyclopedia. Accessed March 23, 2016. http://christiananswers.net/dictionary/onycha.html.

———. "What Are Some of the Most Common Misconceptions about Jesus Christ's Birth?" Accessed March 23, 2016. http://christiananswers.net/christmas /mythsaboutchristmas.html.

Coffman, James Burton. "Coffman's Commentaries on the Bible: Jeremiah 8." StudyLight.org. Accessed March 17, 2016. www.studylight.org/commentaries /bcc/jeremiah-8.html.

Cohen, Suzy. "Dear Pharmacist: How to Make Natural Mosquito Repellent." Orlando Sun-Sentinel. July 6, 2015. Accessed April 2, 2016. www.sun-sentinel.com /health/fl-suzy-cohen-071215-20150706-column.html.

Colon-Rectal.com. "Flatulence, Belching, and Abdominal Gas." Accessed June 22, 2014. http://colon-rectal.com/colon_conditions/gas/.

Dogs Naturally. "Essential Oils for Pets." 2011. Accessed April 4, 2016. www.dogsnaturallymagazine.com/essential-oils-for-pets/.

Drugs.com. "Sandalwood Oil." Accessed March 17, 2016. www.drugs.com/npp /sandalwood-oil.html.

Elaine: Webbed (blog). "Dangerous Essential Oils." http://eethomp.com/AT
/dangerous_oils.html.

Esoteric Oils. "Aniseed Essential Oil Information." Accessed March 17, 2016.
www.essentialoils.co.za/essential-oils/aniseed.htm.

Experience Essential Oils.com. "Cassia Essential Oil: Ancient Bible Oil." Accessed
March 20, 2016. www.experience-essential-oils.com/cassia-essential-oil.html.

———. "Sandalwood Essential Oil Invokes Deep Relaxation, Meditation and More!"
Accessed March 17, 2016. www.experience-essential-oils.com/sandalwood-
essential-oil.html.

———. "The Benefits of Fennel Essential Oil include Supportive to Healthy Digestive
System." Accessed March 17, 2016. www.experience-essential-oils.com/benefits-
of-fennel.html.

Fischer, Melinda, Dr. "Essential Oils to Use While Breastfeeding."
JustBreastFeeding.com. January 17, 2015. Accessed April 4, 2016.
www.justbreastfeeding.com/increasing-breastmilk/essential-oils
-breastfeeding-2/.

Grieve, M. "Aloes." Botanical.com. Accessed March 16, 2016. www.botanical.com
/botanical/mgmh/a/aloes027.html.

Goldman, Rena. "7 Uses for Acacia." HealthLine, November 21, 2014.
www.healthline.com/health/7-uses-for-acacia#1.

Group, Edward. "The Health Benefits of Pine Oil." Global Healing Center.
Last modified October 5, 2015. www.globalhealingcenter.com/natural-health
/pine-oil/.

Guerts, Christine. "Frankincense Essential Oil." The Mountain Rose Blog. August 31,
2012. http://mountainroseblog.com/frankincense-essential-oil/.

Guzik, David. "The Kingdom Parables." Blue Letter Bible. Accessed March 23, 2016.
www.blueletterbible.org/comm/guzik_david/studyguide_mat/mat_13.cfm.

Harris, Lea. "Essential Oils 101: Using Essential Oils for Muscle-Related Pain Relief."
NourishingTreasures.com. March 8, 2013. Accessed June 24, 2014.
www.nourishingtreasures.com/index.php/2013/03/08/essential-oils
-101-using-essential-oils-for-muscle-related-pain-relief/.

Health Benefits Times.com. "Health Benefits of Saffron Essential Oil." Accessed
March 25, 2016. www.healthbenefitstimes.com/health-benefits-saffron
-essential-oil/.

Healthy and Natural World. "The Top 16 Essential Oils to Relieve Pain and
Inflammation." January 13, 2014. Accessed March 25, 2016.
www.healthyandnaturalworld.com/essential-oils-to-relieve-pain/.

Henry, Matthew. "Matthew 13." Matthew Henry Commentary on the Whole Bible.
Accessed March 23, 2016. www.biblestudytools.com/commentaries
/matthew-henry-concise/matthew/13.html.

———. "Song of Solomon 1." Matthew Henry Commentary of the Whole Bible (Concise). BibleStudyTools.com. Accessed March 20, 2016. www.biblestudytools.com/commentaries/matthew-henry-concise /song-of-solomon/song-of-solomon-1.html.

Hermitageoils.com. "Horsemint Organic (Wild Mint)." Accessed March 23, 2016. https://hermitageoils.com/product/horsemint-organic-wild-mint/.

Himalaya Wellness. "Herbal Monograph: Indian Bdellium." Accessed March 16, 2016. www.himalayawellness.com/herbalmonograph/indian-bdellium.htm.

Hodges, Derek. "Pine Essential Oil." AyurvedicOils.com. December 14, 2015. Accessed March 24, 2016. http://ayurvedicoils.com/tag/pinus-pinaster -essential-oil.

———. "Fir Needle Essential Oil." Ayurvedic Oils.com, January 28, 2016. Accessed March 22, 2016. http://ayurvedicoils.com/tag/fir-needle-essential-oil.

Hogan, Rita. "The Dangers of Undiluted Essential Oils for Dogs." Dogs Naturally. March 11, 2016. Accessed April 4, 2016. www.dogsnaturallymagazine.com /dangers-undiluted-essential-oils-dog/.

Hopewell Essential Oils. "Psoriasis." Accessed June 24, 2014. http://hopewelloils. com/psoriasis.php.

Ingredients to Die For. "Rock Rose/Cistus Essential Oil." Accessed March 24, 2016. www.ingredientstodiefor.com/item/Rock_Rose_Cistus_Essential_Oil/1119.

Jabs, Matt. "Simple and Effective Homemade Deodorant." DIY Natural. Accessed June 19, 2014. www.diynatural.com/natural-homemade-deodorant/.

Keay, Penny. "Fatigue Relief Using Essential Oils." Birch Hill Happenings. Accessed June 22, 2014. http://birchhillhappenings.com/fatigue.htm.

———. "Whooping Cough (Pertussis)—Using Essential Oils to Help." Birch Hill Happenings Aromatherapy, LLC. Accessed June 25, 2014. http://birchhillhappenings.com/v1592012whoopingcough.htm.

Keville, Kathi. "Aromatherapy Stress Relief." How Stuff Works. Accessed June 25, 2014. http://health.howstuffworks.com/wellness/natural-medicine /aromatherapy/aromatherapy-stress-relief.htm.

———. "How to Treat Asthma with Aromatherapy." How Stuff Works. Accessed June 18, 2014. http://health.howstuffworks.com/wellness/natural-medicine /aromatherapy/how-to-treat-asthma-with-aromatherapy.htm.

King James Bible Online. Accessed March 14–April 7, 2016. www. kingjamesbibleonline.org.

Ladysessentialsworld. "Need to Know Substitutions for Essential Oils Look Here." Ebay.com. Accessed March 23, 2016. www.ebay.com/gds/Need-to-Know -Substitutions-for-Essential-Oils-Look-Here-/10000000000895330/g.html.

Levy, Gaye. "22 Powerful Uses for Frankincense Essential Oil." Backdoor Survival: Prepping with Optimism. Nov. 21, 2014. Accessed March 22, 2016. www.backdoorsurvival.com/powerful-uses-of-frankincense-essential-oil/.

Life Sciences Publishing. *Essential Oils Desk Reference.* 5th ed., Life Sciences Publishing. 2013.

Low Dog, Tieraona, MD. "3 Ways to Cool Hot Flashes." *Prevention.* July 16, 2013. Accessed June 23, 2014. www.prevention.com/health/health-concerns /natural-remedies-hot-flashes.

McNeal, Erica. "Biblical Oil: Aloes/Sandalwood." Accessed March 17, 2016. www.ericamcneal.com/biblical-oil-used-today-aloessandalwood/.

Mercola, Joseph. "Anise Oil: An Ancient Herbal Wonder." Mercola.com. Accessed March 17, 2016. http://articles.mercola.com/herbal-oils/anise-oil.aspx.

——. "Bay Oil: The Essential Oil for Men." Mercola.com. Accessed March 19, 2016. http://articles.mercola.com/herbal-oils/bay-oil.aspx.

——. "Coriander Seed Oil: More Than Just a Spice." Mercola.com. Accessed March 20, 2016. http://articles.mercola.com/herbal-oils/coriander-seed-oil.aspx.

——. "Pine Oil: A Potential Panacea?" Mercola.com. Accessed March 24, 2016. http://articles.mercola.com/herbal-oils/pine-oil.aspx.

——. "Spearmint Oil: The Gentler Mint Oil." Mercola.com. Accessed March 23, 2016. http://articles.mercola.com/herbal-oils/spearmint-oil.aspx.

Mountain Rose Herbs. "Fir Needle Essential Oil." Accessed March 22, 2016. www.mountainroseherbs.com/products/fir-needle-essential-oil/profile.

——. "Galbanum Essential Oil." Accessed March 22, 2016. www.mountainroseherbs. com/products/galbanum-essential-oil/profile.

Munipalli, Haripriya. "15 Health Benefits of Galbanum Essential Oil." DIY Health Remedies. June 18, 2015. Accessed March 22, 2016. www.diyhealthremedy.com /15-health-benefits-of-galbanum-essential-oil/.

"Natural Diaper Rash Remedy." *Essential Oils for Beginners.* Berkeley, CA: Althea Press, 2013.

Natural Medicinal Herbs. "Medicinal Herbs: Sweet Acacia." Accessed March 25, 2016. www.naturalmedicinalherbs.net/herbs/a/acacia-farnesiana=sweet -acacia.php.

New Health Advisor. "Essential Oil for Arthritis." Accessed March 25, 2016. www.newhealthadvisor.com/Essential-Oils-for-Arthritis.html.

NuKira. "Dangerous Essential Oils." Accessed April 1, 2016. www.nukira.com /pages/dangerous-essential-oils.

Organic Facts. "Health Benefits of Anise Essential Oil." Accessed March 17 & 20, 2016. www.organicfacts.net/health-benefits/essential-oils/health-benefits -of-anise-essential-oil.html.

———. "Health Benefits of Bay Essential Oil." Accessed March 19, 2016. www.organicfacts.net/health-benefits/essential-oils/health-benefits -of-bay-essential-oil.html.

———. "Health Benefits of Calamus Essential Oil." Accessed March 20, 2016. www.organicfacts.net/health-benefits/essential-oils/health-benefits-of -calamus-essential-oil.html.

———. "Health Benefits of Cassia Essential Oil." Accessed March 17 & 20, 2016. www.organicfacts.net/health-benefits/essential-oils/health-benefits-of -cassia-essential-oil.html.

———. "Health Benefits of Cedarwood Essential Oil." Accessed March 20, 2016. www.organicfacts.net/health-benefits/essential-oils/health-benefits-of -cedar-wood-essential-oil.html.

———. "Health Benefits of Cinnamon Oil." Accessed March 20, 2016. www.organicfacts.net/health-benefits/essential-oils/health-benefits -of-cinnamon-oil.html.

———. "Health Benefits of Cumin Essential Oil." Accessed March 21–22, 2016. www.organicfacts.net/health-benefits/essential-oils/health-benefits-of -cumin-essential-oil.html.

———. "Health Benefits of Cypress Essential Oil." Accessed March 22, 2016. www.organicfacts.net/health-benefits/essential-oils/cypress-essential-oil.html.

———. "Health Benefits of Pine Essential Oil." Accessed March 24, 2016. www.organicfacts.net/health-benefits/essential-oils/pine-essential-oil.html.

———. "Health Benefits of Saffron." Accessed March 25, 2016. www.organicfacts.net /health-benefits/herbs-and-spices/saffron.html.

———. "Health Benefits of Sandalwood Essential Oil." Accessed March 17, 2016. www.organicfacts.net/health-benefits/essential-oils/sandalwood-essential -oil.html.

———. "Health Benefits of Spikenard Essential Oil." Accessed March 25, 2016. www.organicfacts.net/health-benefits/essential-oils/health-benefits-of -spikenard-essential-oil.html.

———. "List of Essential Oils." Accessed March 25, 2016. www.organicfacts.net /health-benefits/essential-oils/list-of-essential-oils.html.

———. "List of Essential Oils with their Health Benefits." Accessed March 24, 2016. www.organicfacts.net/health-benefits/essential-oils/list-of-essential-oils.html.

Oshadhi. "Horse Mint Organic, Mentha Longifolia." Accessed March 23, 2016. www.oshadhi.co.uk/horse-mint-organic-mentha-longifolia/.

Palmquist, Richard, Dr. "Pet Aromatherapy and Essential Oils: What You Need To Know." Huffington Post Healthy Living, June 19, 2011. Accessed April 4, 2016. www.huffingtonpost.com/richard-palmquist-dvm/pet-aromatherapy _b_877199.html.

Pedranti, Jo. "Essential Oils that are Adaptogens." Jo's Health Corner. Accessed March 29, 2016. http://joshealthcorner.blogspot.com/2010/01/adaptogens.html.

PharmGKB. "Gene CYP2D6." Accessed March 17, 2016. www.pharmgkb.org/gene /PA128?tabType=tabVip.

Plant Therapy. "Fir Needle Essential Oil." Accessed March 22, 2016. www.planttherapy.com/fir-needle-essential-oil.

Pontillo, Rachel. "How to Holistically Prevent and Heal Chapped Lips." Holistically Haute. December 13, 2012. Accessed June 19, 2014. www.holisticallyhaute.com /2012/12/how-to-holistically-prevent-and-heal-chapped-lips-plus-a-special -treat.html.

Power, Dr. Joie. "Artisan Essential Oils: Balsam Poplar Oil." The Aromatherapy School. Accessed March 17, 2016. www.aromatherapy-school.com/essential-oils /balsam-poplar-essential-oil.html.

Rayma, Maria. "A Guide to Essential Oil Substitutions." Humblebee & Me. August 5, 2013. Accessed March 20, 2016. www.humblebeeandme.com/a-guide-to -essential-oil-substitutions/.

Rodriguez, Tori. "Essential Oils Might Be the New Antibiotics." The Atlantic, January 16, 2015. Accessed March 29, 2016. www.theatlantic.com/health /archive/2015/01/the-new-antibiotics-might-be-essential-oils/384247/.

Ross, Allen. "3. The Visit of the Wise Men (Matthew 2:1–12)." Bible.org. Accessed March 23, 2016. https://bible.org/seriespage/3-visit-wise-men-matthew-21-12.

Ryman, Danièle. "Bay Tree." Aromatherapy Bible. Accessed March 19, 2016. http://aromatherapybible.com/bay-tree/.

———. "Cedarwood." Aromatherapy Bible. Accessed March 20, 2016. http://aromatherapybible.com/cedarwood/.

———. "Galbanum." Aromatherapy Bible. Accessed March 22, 2016. http://aromatherapybible.com/galbanum/.

———. "Laurel." Aromatherapy Bible. Accessed March 19, 2016. http://aromatherapybible.com/laurel/.

Schulman, Jennifer. "Adaptogens: What are They? How Do They Benefit our Health? Where Can We Get Them?" JenniferSchulman.com. Accessed March 29, 2016. www.jenniferschulman.com/adaptogens.

Sonoma Press. Essential Oils and Aromatherapy: An Introductory Guide. Berkeley, CA: Sonoma Press, 2014.

Steinbrinck, Kasey. "Facts about Frankincense and Myrrh and How They Affect Your Health." Natural Healthy Concepts, December 24, 2013. Accessed March 22, 2016. http://blog.naturalhealthyconcepts.com/2013/12/24/facts-frankincense-myrrh/.

Stillpoint Aromatics. "Balsam Poplar Essential Oil." Accessed March 17, 2016. www.stillpointaromatics.com/balsam-poplar-Populus-balsamifera-essential-oil.

———. "Cistus (Rock Rose) Essential Oil." Accessed March 24, 2016. www.stillpointaromatics.com/cistus-rock-rose-Cistus-ladaniferus -essential-oil-aromatherapy.

StudyLight.org. "Verse-by-Verse Bible Commentary: Song of Solomon." Accessed March 20, 2016. www.studylight.org/commentary/song-of-solomon/.

Sustainable Baby Steps. "Coriander Essential Oil: Uses, Benefits and Precautions." Accessed March 20, 2016. www.sustainablebabysteps.com/coriander-essential -oil.html.

———. "Cypress Essential Oil: Uses, Benefits and Precautions." Accessed March 22, 2016. www.sustainablebabysteps.com/cypress-oil.html.

The Epistle. "God Will Save Me." Accessed March 29, 2016. http://epistle.us /inspiration/godwillsaveme.html.

United States Conference of Catholic Bishops. "Psalms, Chapter 37." Accessed March 19, 2016. www.usccb.org/bible/psalms/37.

Victorie. "Acacia (Shittim) Absolute." Accessed March 25, 2016. www.victorie-inc.us/acacia.html.

———. "Myrtle, Red." Accessed March 23, 2016. www.victorie-inc.us/myrtle.html.

Webb, Becky. "2 Essential Oils that May Maintain Healthy Milk Production in Nursing Mothers." Rooted Blessings, October 27, 2013. Accessed April 4, 2016. www.rootedblessings.com/2-essential-oils-that-increase-milk-production -in-nursing-mothers/.

WildLebanon.org. "Pine Forest." Accessed March 24, 2016. www.wildlebanon.org /en/pages/hab/pineforest.html.

Worwood, Valerie Ann. *The Complete Book of Essential Oils and Aromatherapy*. New World Library, 1991; Kindle edition.

Wycliffe Associates. "Waiting for God: Psalm 37." Accessed March 19, 2016. www.easyenglish.info/psalms/psalm037-taw.htm.

Young, Gary D. "12 Oils of Ancient Scripture: Sandalwood." D. Gary Young's Blog. January 5, 2010. www.dgaryyoung.com/blog/2010/12-oils-of-ancient-scripture -sandalwood/.

Young Living Essential Oils. "Age Spots and Essential Oils." Accessed June 22, 2014. www.pinterest.com/pin/189854940516175623/.

———. "Cedarwood Essential Oil." Accessed March 17, 2016. www.youngliving.com /en_US/products/cedarwood-essential-oil.

———. "Coriander Essential Oil." Accessed March 20, 2016. www.youngliving.com /en_US/products/coriander-essential-oil.

———. "Galbanum Essential Oil." Accessed March 17, 2016. www.youngliving.com
/en_US/products/galbanum-essential-oil.

Zappia, Anthony. "15 Essential Oils for Stress Relief." WellBeing.com. May 1, 2013.
Accessed March 29, 2016. www.wellbeing.com.au/blog/15-essential-oils-for
-stress-relief/.

Acknowledgments

EVERY BOOK IS a joyful collaboration among many team members, and a book about essential oils and Bible verse lends itself naturally to this. It has truly been a pleasure working with such an enthusiastic and skilled team of creative folks.

I must thank my friends and colleagues at Althea Press, including my editor, Stacy Wagner-Kinnear, who invited me to participate in this project and provided so much of her knowledgeable guidance and experience. Development editor Mary Cassells and copy editor Meredith Tennant turned the manuscript into a book, while illustrator Tom Bingham brought the Bible's most fragrant plants to life. Designer Adam Johnson brought shape, consistency, and style to this volume, and production manager Kim Ciabattari magically kept the entire process on track. I know there are many more people behind the scenes who should be acknowledged, but authors rarely meet all of these good souls—so I simply thank them for all of their meticulous attention and fine work.

On the spiritual side, I thank Deacon Georgia Carney of the Episcopal Diocese of Rochester, New York, for the information she provided about the modern use of anointment in the Christian faith. The friends and family who are part of my spiritual life are too numerous to mention, but they have been with me throughout this exploration—and will continue to be part of my journey through this life.

Finally, I thank the readers who join me in embracing the natural world and all of the remarkable things in it, whether you indulge in the use of essential oils or take in the wonders of nature in the fields, forests, mountain ranges, seashores, and parks from Acadia to Zion. May you continue to delight in what we find outside, even as you make the most of what we have inside.

About the Author

RANDI MINETOR is the author of more than 50 books on nature, travel, psychology, and medical and general interest topics, with broad expertise in native wildflowers and gardening. A perpetual scholar raised in the Western Judeo-Christian tradition, she studied the Bible in depth as part of her university education, and continues to pursue a spiritual life and a personal relationship with God. Among her essential oils publications is the Sonoma Press bestseller, *Essential Oils and Aromatherapy: An Introductory Guide.* She lives in Rochester, NY.

Index of Ailments and Remedies

Index

CPSIA information can be obtained
at www.ICGtesting.com
Printed in the USA
JSHW041113291020
9218JS00010B/196